35 Day Chakra Journal

A 35 Day Practice For Balancing Your Chakras & Allowing Light, Healing & Happiness Into Your Life

Jenny Douglas

contents

JENNY DOUGLAS

This one's for Vanessa
co-conspirator in all things woo

INTRODUCTION

W elcome, dear reader, to a transformative journey of self-discovery and healing. In this book, we will explore the ancient wisdom of the chakra system and how it can be harnessed to cultivate balance, harmony, and vitality in every aspect of your life By understanding and working with the seven main energy centres of the body, you can unlock your full potential and experience a profound sense of connection to yourself, others, and the world around you.

Chakras are the energy centres of the body. There are seven main chakras, and many minor ones, and between the chakras run many thousands of *nadis*, or energetic channels. In this book, we will focus on the most commonly known chakras. You probably know of chakras as part of an ancient energy system known as prana, or life force, in Hindu and Buddhist beliefs, and these days they are widely known across the Western world as well. Whilst Buddhism holds that there are four main chakras, we are going to use the traditional Hindu designation of seven.

Our chakras are part of the subtle body. While we are aware of our physical body taking up mass in the visual universe, the subtle body comprises energy and mind, and we have to turn a little inward to sense it. The physical and subtle bodies are intimately linked; if there is a disturbance in one field, the effects will also be felt in the other. Happily, this means that when we address the needs of our subtle, energetic body, our physical body will also benefit!

When healthy, each chakra is a spinning disc of energy, distributing energy to its associated area. You feel balanced, at ease in your own body, comfortable within your life. When our chakras are balanced and functioning optimally, we feel grounded, creative, confident, loving, expressive, intuitive, and spiritually connected.

When unhealthy, a chakra may spin too fast or stop moving altogether. Whether a chakra is blocked or overactive, you will see corresponding physical and emotional issues with the region associated with the unhealthy chakra. You may feel wired or sluggish, angry or tearful, struggle to think clearly, to have healthy relationships, or to move or behave in the ways that you know would be most beneficial for you. When our chakras become blocked or imbalanced, we often experience not only physical ailments, but emotional distress, mental cloudiness, and a sense of disconnection from our true selves.

In today's fast-paced, over-stimulated, and often stressful world, it is all too easy for our chakras to become misaligned. We may find ourselves feeling anxious, depleted, or stuck in negative patterns of thought and behaviour. The good news is that by engaging in practices that support and nurture our chakras, we can restore balance and flow to our energy system, allowing us to live with greater ease, joy, and purpose.

You may have some idea of where you are unbalanced, or you may have no idea where to start! Either is fine. If you already know which of your chakras needs attention, jump directly to that section and dive in. If you just feel generally out of sorts, you're in the right place. Congratulate yourself for honouring your need to take care of your whole self – body, mind, and spirit – and go gently into the next 35 days, taking one day at a time, and carrying any new knowledge that resonates with you on into the rest of your life.

In the following pages, you will find many different ways of balancing each chakra, giving you tools to experiment with. Each of these modalities offers a unique pathway to healing and transformation. These modalities include journaling, yoga, EFT (Emotional Freedom Technique), meditation, crystals, physical activities, and foods. By incorporating these practices into your daily life, you can create a powerful toolkit for self-care and personal growth. Let's explore them a little more now.

Journaling is a simple yet profound practice that allows you to connect with your inner world and explore your thoughts, feelings, and experiences in a safe and non-judgmental space. By the simple act of putting pen to paper, you can gain clarity, insight, and perspective on the issues that may be blocking or disrupting your chakras. Each chapter of this book includes journaling prompts and exercises designed to help you dive deep into the energy of each chakra and uncover the wisdom that lies within. Don't overthink it as you write! You're not writing for anyone's eyes but your own. Don't self-edit or censor yourself. You can write in a gorgeous notebook if you like, or on the back of an envelope that you're going to recycle, or even choose a piece of paper you can then ceremoniously burn! It's up to you; there is no wrong way to journal.

Yoga is another powerful tool for balancing the chakras. This ancient practice combines physical postures, breathing techniques, and meditation to promote flexibility, strength, and relaxation in the body and mind. By practicing yoga regularly, you can release tension, improve circulation, and cultivate a sense of inner peace and wellbeing. Each chapter of this book includes yoga postures and sequences specifically designed to target and balance each chakra. Please remember that yoga is not a competitive sport! It doesn't matter how flexible you are, how strong you are, whether you've practiced yoga daily for years or this is your first time trying it. You might find that one day, a pose is easy, and the next time you try it, it feels impossible! Either, and anywhere on the scale between, is fine. Yoga is about being in the now, just you and your body. Nothing else matters except htat you are listening to your body as you move it.

EFT, or Emotional Freedom Technique, is a form of energy psychology that involves tapping on specific acupressure points while focusing on a particular issue or emotion. This practice has been shown to be effective in reducing stress, anxiety, and emotional distress, and can be a powerful tool for clearing blockages in the chakras. Each chapter of this book includes EFT scripts and exercises tailored to the energy of each chakra, and the instructions are repeated for each chakra. Once you get the hang of EFT it is an incredibly portable tool! Memorise the pattern, and you can take it everywhere you go. It's like having a therapist in your pocket! You can adapt the EFT scripts to anything you like, remembering to acknowledge the way you feel right now, even when it is 'negative' – always allow your feelings space to breathe. I quite often tap in the car – it takes some practice and I'm sure other drivers at the red lights wonder what I'm doing, but it's a great way of working out discomfort in the safety of my own company.

Meditation is a foundational practice for balancing the chakras and cultivating inner peace and clarity. By sitting in stillness and focusing on the breath, a mantra, or a visualisation, you can quiet the mind, connect with your inner wisdom, and experience a sense of unity and wholeness. Each chapter of this book includes guided meditations and visualisation exercises designed to activate and balance each chakra. Lots of people believe that they can't 'do' meditation, that sitting still and quiet just isn't possible for them, but this is another non-competitive activity. One day you might sit for five whole minutes in complete peace, whilst another day you may feel fidgety after two, and your thoughts are scattered and jumping around in your head. The strongest advice I can give you is this: when your thoughts pop up (and they will), just observe them, and let them go. That s it! Don't judge yourself, don't assume that other people can do it 'perfectly,' and when (not if!) the thoughts take your attention, just notice, and bring yourself back to neutrality. There is no wrong way to do this.

Guided meditation is an excellent way to start meditating, and you can begin with very short meditations. You do not need to sit for an hour! Five minutes is fine! Five minutes a day will still work wonders for your mental and spiritual health, so I encourage you to persevere. There are plenty of guided meditations available online, and lots of different apps. I am a meditation teacher on the app Insight Timer, and I have lots of free meditations there that you can try.

Crystals have been used for centuries as tools for healing and spiritual growth. Each crystal has its own unique energy signature and can be used to support and amplify the energy of the chakras. By placing crystals on or near the body, or simply holding them during meditation or yoga practice, you can tap into their healing properties and promote balance and harmony in your energy system. Each chapter of this book includes recommendations for crystals that resonate with each chakra. A whole book could be written (and many have) on the energetic qualities of different crystals. If crystals don't resonate energetically with you, that's fine. You can use them as a point of focus during your meditations, or simply disregard them all together. If you have a particalar crystal that you do really resonate with, but it's not listed on the chakra page, that's fine too! Trust your own energy.

Physical activities such as walking, dancing, and martial arts can also be powerful tools for balancing the chakras. These activities help to move energy through the body, release tension and blockages, and promote a sense of vitality and aliveness. Each chapter of this book includes suggestions for physical activities that can support the health and balance of each chakra. If daily life feels overwhelming and you're not sure how to fit an extra physical activity in, don't panic or put pressure on yourself. The smallest acts of mindful movement are still so good for you. Being conscious of your body as you walk up the stairs, breathing the fresh air on your way to the car, having a little dance in the kitchen while the kettle boils – all of these help to keep the energy flowing through our bodies.

Finally, **the foods we eat** can have a profound impact on the health and balance of our chakras. Each chakra is associated with specific colours, elements, and organs in the body, and by consuming foods that resonate with these energies, we can promote balance and vitality in our energy system. Each chapter of this book includes recommendations for foods that support each chakra. Use your creativity to put together dishes that fill you with happiness and fulfilment as you eat them! Enjoy your food in the knowledge that you are benefit your internal energy system on all levels.

And so to conclude. As we journey through the seven main chakras together, from the root chakra at the base of the spine to the crown chakra at the top of the head, we will explore the unique qualities and challenges of each energy centre. We will discover how imbalances in each chakra can manifest in our physical, emotional, and spiritual lives, and how we can use the modalities of journaling, yoga, EFT, meditation, crystals, physical activities, and foods to restore balance and harmony. We will end up happier, healthier, calmer, more able to withstand bumps and swerves in the road, and with a greater depth of knowledge and self-awareness to take onward with us.

Profound transformations can occur when we commit to a practice of regular chakra balancing. By incorporating these modalities into our daily lives, we can cultivate a deep sense of harmony, vitality, and purpose, and unlock our full potential as spiritual beings having a human experience. Remember, the journey of chakra balancing is not a destination, but a lifelong practice of self-discovery, healing, and growth. Each day presents new opportunities to connect with our inner wisdom, release old patterns and blockages, and align ourselves with the flow of universal energy. By committing to this practice, we not only transform ourselves but also contribute to the healing and evolution of the world around us.

So, my friend, I invite you to approach this journey with an open heart and a curious mind. Maybe you already know that yoga is a great fit for you, or maybe crystals are something new that you haven't really played with before. Whichever stage of self-discovery you're at, trust in the wisdom of your own body and soul, and know that you have everything you need within you to create a life of balance, joy, and purpose. Seven chakras, five days for each chakra, and every day a different activity and journal prompt. By the end of this 35 day practice, you will have delved into your own deepest self and rebalanced yourself from root to crown.

May this book be a trusted companion and guide on your path of self-discovery and transformation, and may you become and remain peaceful, balanced and whole.

With love and blessings,

Jenny

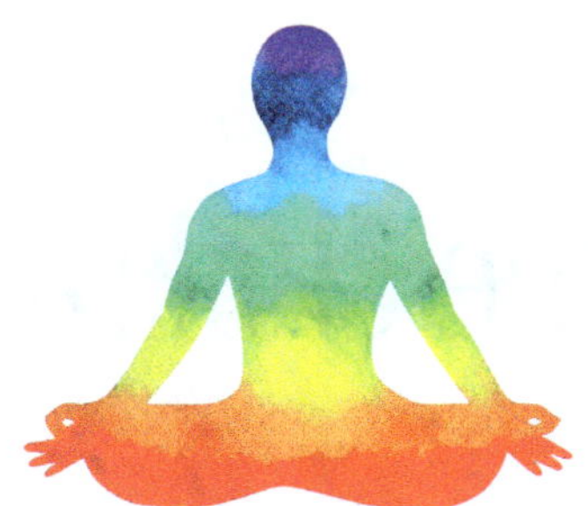

THE CHAKRAS

The first chakra we will explore is the root chakra, or Muladhara, which is located at the base of the spine and is associated with the element of earth. This chakra governs our sense of safety, security, and belonging, and when it is balanced, we feel grounded, stable, and connected to our physical reality. However, when the root chakra is blocked or imbalanced, we may experience feelings of fear, anxiety, and insecurity, as well as physical symptoms such as digestive issues or lower back pain.

To balance the root chakra, we will explore practices such as grounding yoga postures, journaling prompts that help us connect with our sense of safety and security, and EFT exercises that release fears and anxieties. We will also work with crystals such as red jasper and black tourmaline, which are known for their grounding and protective properties, and explore physical activities such as walking barefoot in nature or practicing martial arts to cultivate a sense of stability and strength. Finally, we will discover foods that resonate with the root chakra, such as root vegetables, protein-rich foods, and red-coloured fruits and vegetables.

 As we move up the body to the sacral chakra, or Svadhisthana, we will explore the energy of creativity, sensuality, and emotional flow. This chakra is associated with the element of water and governs our ability to experience pleasure, joy, and abundance. When the sacral chakra is balanced, we feel creative, passionate, and emotionally vibrant, but when it is blocked or imbalanced, we may experience feelings of shame, guilt, or emotional numbness, as well as physical symptoms such as reproductive issues or lower back pain.

To balance the sacral chakra, we will explore practices such as hip-opening yoga postures, journaling prompts that help us connect with our creative and sensual nature, and EFT exercises that release emotional blockages and traumas. We will also work with crystals such as orange calcite and carnelian, which are known for their energising and creativity-enhancing properties, and explore physical activities such as dancing or swimming to cultivate a sense of fluidity and grace. Finally, we will discover foods that resonate with the sacral chakra, such as tropical fruits, nuts and seeds, and orange-coloured foods.

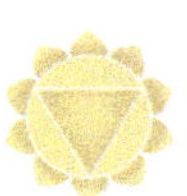 As we continue our journey up the body, we will explore the solar plexus chakra, or Manipura, which is associated with the element of fire and governs our sense of personal power, self-esteem, and identity. When this chakra is balanced, we feel confident, assertive, and in control of our lives, but when it is blocked or imbalanced, we may experience feelings of shame, self-doubt, and powerlessness, as well as physical symptoms such as digestive issues or fatigue.

To balance the solar plexus chakra, we will explore practices such as core-strengthening yoga postures, journaling prompts that help us connect with our inner strength and purpose, and EFT exercises that release limiting beliefs and self-doubts. We will also work with crystals such as citrine and pyrite, which are known for their energising and confidence-boosting properties, and explore physical activities such as running or martial arts to cultivate a sense of personal power and vitality. Finally, we will discover foods that resonate with the solar plexus chakra, such as yellow-coloured foods, spices, and complex carbohydrates.

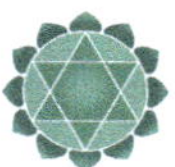

As we move into the heart chakra, or Anahata, we will explore the energy of love, compassion, and relationships. This chakra is associated with the element of air and governs our ability to give and receive love, both for ourselves and others. When the heart chakra is balanced, we feel open, loving, and connected to the world around us, but when it is blocked or imbalanced, we may experience feelings of loneliness, grief, or difficulty in relationships, as well as physical symptoms such as chest pain or respiratory issues.

To balance the heart chakra, we will explore practices such as heart-opening yoga postures, journaling prompts that help us cultivate self-love and compassion, and EFT exercises that release emotional wounds and promote forgiveness. We will also work with crystals such as rose quartz and green aventurine, which are known for their healing and nurturing properties, and explore physical activities such as hiking or volunteering to cultivate a sense of connection and purpose. Finally, we will discover foods that resonate with the heart chakra, such as leafy greens, green tea, and herbs like basil and thyme.

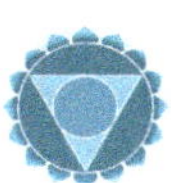

As we continue our journey up the body, we will explore the throat chakra, or Vishuddha, which is associated with the element of ether and governs our ability to communicate our truth and express ourselves authentically. When this chakra is balanced, we feel confident in our self-expression and able to speak our truth with clarity and integrity, but when it is blocked or imbalanced, we may experience feelings of shyness, difficulty in communication, or a fear of speaking up, as well as physical symptoms such as throat pain or thyroid issues.

To balance the throat chakra, we will explore practices such as throat-opening yoga postures, journaling prompts that help us find our authentic voice and express our truth, and EFT exercises that release fears and blockages around communication. We will also work with crystals such as blue lace agate and sodalite, which are known for their calming and truth-enhancing properties, and explore physical activities such as singing or chanting to cultivate a sense of creative self-expression. Finally, we will discover foods that resonate with the throat chakra, such as fruits like blueberries and blackberries, herbal teas, and foods with a high water content.

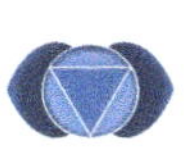

As we move into the third eye chakra, or Ajna, we will explore the energy of intuition, insight, and spiritual vision. This chakra is associated with the element of light and governs our ability to see beyond the physical world and connect with our inner wisdom and guidance. When the third eye chakra is balanced, we feel intuitive, imaginative, and spiritually connected, but when it is blocked or imbalanced, we may experience feelings of confusion, lack of direction, or difficulty in trusting our intuition, as well as physical symptoms such as headaches or vision problems.

To balance the third eye chakra, we will explore practices such as meditation and visualisation exercises, journaling prompts that help us connect with our inner guidance and wisdom, and EFT exercises that release limiting beliefs and mental blockages. We will also work with crystals such as amethyst and lapis lazuli, which are known for their intuitive and spiritually uplifting properties, and explore physical activities such as yoga or tai chi to cultivate a sense of inner focus and clarity. Finally, we will discover foods that resonate with the third eye chakra, such as purple-coloured foods, dark chocolate, and herbal teas like lavender and chamomile.

 Finally, as we reach the crown chakra, or Sahasrara, at the top of the head, we will explore the energy of spiritual connection, enlightenment, and unity consciousness. This chakra is associated with the element of pure consciousness and governs our ability to connect with the divine and experience a sense of oneness with all that is. When the crown chakra is balanced, we feel a deep sense of inner peace, spiritual connection, and a knowing that we are part of something greater than ourselves, but when it is blocked or imbalanced, we may experience feelings of disconnection, spiritual emptiness, or a lack of purpose, as well as physical symptoms such as depression or a sense of being ungrounded.

To balance the crown chakra, we will explore practices such as meditation and prayer, journaling prompts that help us connect with our higher self and spiritual purpose, and EFT exercises that release any remaining blockages or limitations in our energy system. We will also work with crystals such as clear quartz and selenite, which are known for their spiritually elevating and purifying properties, and explore physical activities such as yoga or walking in nature to cultivate a sense of unity and connection with the world around us. Finally, we will discover foods that resonate with the crown chakra, such as foods that are light and pure, like fresh fruits and vegetables, as well as herbal teas and pure water.

ROOT

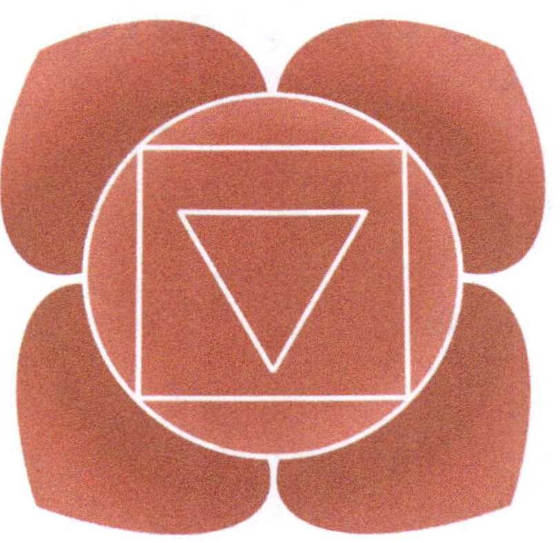

I am

ROOT Chakra

ROOT

Chakra Number: 1
Element: Earth
Colour: Red
Sound: LAM

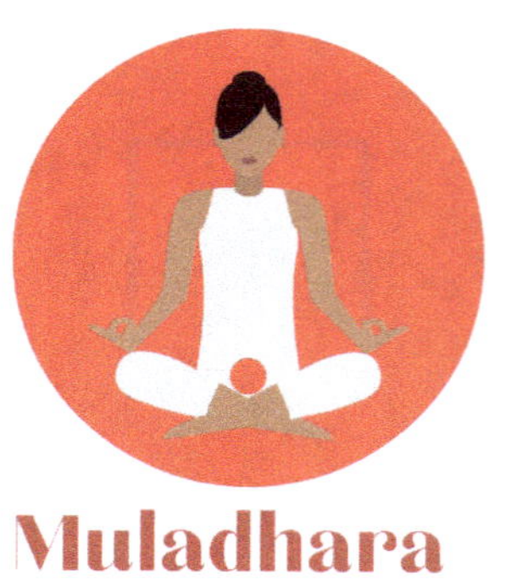

Muladhara

The root chakra is the foundational energy centre, and is located at the base of the spine. Its symbol is a deep red lotus flower with four petals, and its element is earth. It represents our foundations, our sense of stability and security, and our connection to the physical world. The root chakra is associated with feelings of safety, being grounded, and our survival instincts. It also governs such aspects as our sense of belonging, trust, and our ability to meet basic needs. Balancing and nurturing this chakra can help promote a sense of stability in our bodies and in our lives, and gives us a solid foundation for a general sense of wellbeing.

Symptoms of an Overactive Root Chakra

Anger / short temper

Belligerence

Impatience

Back pain

Digestive difficulties

Feeling of heaviness

Feeling of wanting

Never feeling satisfied

Symptoms of an Underactive Root Chakra

Sense of insecurity

Spaced out & dreamy

Disconnected from reality

Anxiety & worry

Painful periods

Depression

Frustration

Lack of energy & fatigue

ROOT DAY 1: PHYSICAL ACTIVITY

We'll start our 35 day practice here at the root chakra, with some physical activity to support and nurture the Muldhara. This foundational energy centre is associated with our sense of grounding, stability, and connection to the earth. When the root chakra is balanced, we feel secure, centred, and able to navigate the challenges of life with ease and grace.

Engaging in physical activities that connect us to the earth and to our bodies is a powerful way to cultivate this sense of grounding and stability. The simple act of moving our bodies mindfully and with intention helps release stagnant energy and blockages in the root chakra, allowing us to feel more rooted, present, and alive.

The most obvious grounding exercise is also the easiest, and it's free! Depending on the time of year, of course, since you might not want to do this in the depths of winter in the northern hemisphere, but this activity shows you how simple practices can have a profound effect. This physical activity is, of course, getting your skin onto the earth.

Walking barefoot on the earth is deeply nourishing for the root chakra. Known as "earthing" or "grounding," this practice involves direct contact between the soles of our feet and the natural surfaces of the earth, such as grass, sand, or soil. By connecting with the earth in this way, we allow its stabilising, healing energy to flow into our bodies, promoting a sense of balance and well-being. Being barefoot on the earth can be especially beneficial for those who spend much of their day indoors or disconnected from nature. The simple act of removing our shoes and feeling the ground beneath our feet can help to discharge any accumulated stress or tension, allowing us to reconnect with the natural world and our own inner sense of grounding. A similar effect can be found in gardening with bare hands – no gardening gloves! By getting your fingers and palms directly into the soil – even in a pot or windowsill container – you are connecting with earth energy, and activating all the senses that are part of millennia of biological heritage. We are designed to be in touch with mother Earth.

Gardening in any way you can is incredibly nourishing for the root chakra. By getting our hands dirty and connecting with the earth, we cultivate a sense of patience, nurturing, and growth. As we plant seeds, tend to our gardens, and watch our efforts bear fruit, we develop a deep appreciation for the cycles of life and the abundance of the natural world. This connection to the earth can be incredibly stabilising, reminding us of our own inherent worth and the importance of tending to our own needs with love and care.

Another activity that can be incredibly beneficial for the root chakra is the practice of martial arts. Not what you were expecting, right?! Disciplines such as karate, taekwondo, and aikido not only provide a full-body workout but also help to cultivate a deep sense of inner strength, confidence, and resilience. When we move through the powerful stances and techniques of these ancient practices, we connect with our inner warrior, learning to stand our ground and defend ourselves both physically and emotionally.

The martial arts also teach us the importance of being present and grounded in the moment. By focusing our attention on our breath, our movements, and our opponent, we develop a keen sense of awareness and concentration, anchoring us firmly in the here and now. This mindfulness can be incredibly valuable in our daily lives, helping us to stay centred and calm in the face of stress or adversity. Taking a martial arts class is best done through a professional organisation and it may not be something you want to or are able to do right now, but perhaps a practice like tai chi, with its slow, intentional movements, can offer an insight into this kind of physical wisdom. Tai chi or qu gong are both wonderful tools for balancing the root chakra. Their gentle, flowing movements help to circulate energy throughout the body whilst also promoting a sense of grounding and stability. As you move through the postures and focus on your breath, you cultivate a deep sense of inner peace and harmony, allowing you to feel more rooted and centred in your daily life. If you're curious about either of these there are tons of free videos available online, and if you feel called to, take a class! It might change your life.

Decluttering your physical space can have a profound impact on the root chakra. Clutter and disorganisation creates a sense of chaos and instability in your environment, which can translate into feelings of unease and disconnection from your surroundings. By removing unnecessary items and creating a clean, orderly space, you can cultivate a sense of control and mastery over your physical reality, which is essential for a balanced root chakra. Moreover, the act of decluttering itself can be a grounding and empowering experience. As you sort through your belongings and make decisions about what to keep and what to let go of, you're actively engaging with your physical world and asserting your autonomy. This process can help to strengthen your sense of self and reinforce your connection to the present moment, both of which are crucial for a healthy root chakra.

As you explore these various physical activities, remember that the key to balancing the root chakra is to find practices that resonate with you personally. What makes *you* feel grounded, secure, and connected to your body and the earth? Trust your intuition and allow yourself to be guided towards the activities that nourish you on a deep level.

It's also important to approach these practices with mindfulness and self-compassion. Rather than pushing yourself to achieve a certain goal or outcome, focus on the journey itself, allowing each moment to unfold with curiosity and acceptance. If you find yourself getting caught up in self-judgment or comparison, gently redirect your attention back to your breath and the sensations in your body, reminding yourself that you are exactly where you need to be. This isn't a competition!

As you incorporate these physical activities into your daily life, you'll find that your root chakra begins to feel more balanced and harmonised. You may notice a greater sense of stability, security, and groundedness, both in your physical body and your emotional landscape. You may also find that you are better able to handle the ups and downs of life, trusting in your own resilience and the support of the earth beneath your feet.

Choose One of the Following Activities

Mindful Walking

Go for a mindful walk, either outside in nature or simply around your neighbourhood. As you walk, bring your attention to the sensation of your feet making contact with the ground. Notice the rhythm of your steps and the feeling of your muscles working to propel you forward. If it's safe and appropriate to do so, go barefoot!

As you continue to walk, expand your awareness to include the sights, sounds, and smells around you. Notice the colours of the leaves, the chirping of the birds, and the scent of the fresh air. Allow yourself to be fully present in the moment, letting go of any worries or distractions and simply enjoying the simple act of moving your body through space.

If your mind begins to wander, gently redirect your attention back to your feet and your surroundings. Remind yourself that this walk is an opportunity to connect with your body and the world around you, grounding yourself in the present moment.

Gardening

Take yourself into your garden, find a community gardening project, or get an indoor plant pot or container. Spend some time in a gardening activity that involves getting your hands in the soil. Plant some seeds, do some weeding, or prepare a flower or vegetable bed. If it's the middle of winter, either tend to your houseplants (or buy a houseplant to care for), plant some bulbs for next spring's flowers, or simply wrap up warm, take a thick blanket, and go and sit outside for ten minutes of mindful mediation, as connected to the earth as you can be.

Martial Arts

Research a local class and see if there are any martial arts taht you could learn that would strengthen your connection to your root chakra. If this isn't an option, find some online videos delivered by reputable teachers, and do a physical session it he comfort of your home. Remember, it's about being connected to your body as you are led through each movement.

Decluttering

Give yourself the luxury of a clear space in your home, even if it is only a shelf or one single drawer. Decluttering helps to release emotional and energetic blockages that might be associated with certain objects or areas of one's home. By letting go of items that no longer serve you or that carry negative associations, you're creating space for new, positive energy to flow into your life! This applies to mental, emotional, and spiritual decluttering too. This might look like spending time deleting emails that you no longer need to keep, unfollowing social media accounts that you no longer resonate with, or acknowledging and releasing limiting beliefs that no longer serve you. Any or all of these will make space for new, positive energy to take root and flourish.

ROOT Day 1: Journal Prompt

What does stability mean to you in various areas of your life, such as relationships, work, and personal well-being? Reflect on moments when you felt most stable and grounded. What factors contributed to that sense of stability?

ROOT Day 2: Foods, Drinks, Herbs & Spices

Just as physical activities can help to ground and stabilise us, the nourishment we provide for our bodies can play a crucial role in promoting a sense of vitality, security, and connection to the earth. Our bodies are our homes, where we come back to to find ourselves, and our bodies are always with us! Taking care of your body can be a joy.

When the root chakra is in balance, we feel a strong sense of safety, stability, and groundedness in our physical body. We have a healthy relationship with food, seeing it as a source of nourishment and pleasure rather than a source of stress or anxiety. We are able to trust in the abundance of the earth, as well as our own ability to meet our basic needs.

To support this sense of balance and harmony in the root chakra, it's important to focus on foods that are grounding, nourishing, and sustaining. These foods tend to be rich in protein, healthy fats, and complex carbohydrates, providing a slow and steady release of energy that can help to keep us feeling centred and focused throughout the day.

One of the key components of a root chakra-balancing diet is an emphasis on whole, unprocessed foods. These foods are typically closer to their natural state, retaining more of their inherent nutrients and life force energy. When we eat whole foods, we are essentially consuming the vitality and grounding energy of the earth itself, allowing us to feel more connected to the natural world and our own physical body.

Some specific whole foods that can be particularly nourishing for the root chakra include:

Root vegetables: As their name suggests, root vegetables such as potatoes, carrots, beetroot, and parsnips are deeply grounding and nourishing. They grow beneath the surface of the earth, absorbing its stabilising energy and nutrients. When we eat these vegetables, we are essentially taking in this grounding energy, helping to anchor us in the present moment and provide a sense of stability and security.

Protein-rich foods: Protein is essential for building and repairing tissues in the body, and it can also help to promote feelings of satiety and grounding. Good sources of protein for the root chakra include lean meats, fish, eggs, beans, lentils, and tofu. These foods provide a slow and steady release of energy, helping to keep us feeling balanced and sustained throughout the day.

Healthy fats: Like protein, healthy fats can help to promote feelings of satiety and grounding. They also play a crucial role in hormone production and brain function, supporting overall physical and emotional well-being. Good sources of healthy fats include avocados, nuts, seeds, olive oil, and fatty fish like salmon and sardines.

Whole grains: Complex carbohydrates, like whole grains, provide a slow and steady release of energy, helping to keep us feeling grounded and focused. Good options include brown rice, quinoa, oats, and whole grain bread. These foods are also rich in fibre, which can help to promote healthy digestion and elimination.

Red foods: In chakra theory, the colour red is associated with the root chakra. Eating foods that are naturally red in colour, such as apples, beets, cherries, and red bell peppers, can help to stimulate and balance this energy centre. These foods are also rich in antioxidants and other nutrients that support overall health and vitality.

In addition to these specific foods, it's important to focus on eating a wide variety of colourful fruits and vegetables. These foods are packed with vitamins, minerals, and other nutrients that support overall health and well-being, promoting a sense of vitality and connection to the earth.

When it comes to drinks, water is perhaps the most important substance for balancing the root chakra. Water is essential for maintaining proper hydration, flushing toxins from the body, and promoting healthy digestion and elimination. Aim to drink at least 8 glasses of water per day, or more if you are physically active or live in a hot climate.

Other drinks that can be supportive of the root chakra include herbal teas, particularly those made with grounding roots like ginger, turmeric, and dandelion. These teas can help to promote a sense of warmth and stability in the body, while also providing a host of other health benefits.

It's also important to be mindful of the *way* we eat and drink, not just what we consume. When we eat in a rushed or distracted state, we are less likely to fully appreciate and absorb the nourishment we are taking in. We may also be more likely to overeat or make less healthy food choices.

To support mindful eating and drinking, try to create a peaceful and pleasant environment for your meals. Sit down at a table, away from distractions like television or electronics. Take a moment to express gratitude for the food and the people who helped to bring it to your plate. Engage your senses fully, noticing the colours, smells, and textures of your food.

As you eat, take your time and chew each bite thoroughly. Pay attention to the flavours and sensations in your mouth, savouring each morsel. Notice how your body feels as you eat, tuning in to your hunger and fullness cues. Allow yourself to stop eating when you feel satisfied, even if there is still food on your plate.

By bringing mindfulness and intention to our eating and drinking habits, we can cultivate a deeper sense of connection to our bodies and the nourishment we are taking in. We can learn to trust our own internal wisdom, making food choices that support our individual needs and preferences.

Of course, it's important to remember that everyone's dietary needs are different, and what works for one person may not work for another. If you have specific health concerns or dietary restrictions, it's always best to consult with a qualified healthcare provider or registered dietitian to develop a plan that is tailored to your individual needs. It's also important to be gentle with yourself and avoid getting too caught up in the idea of a "perfect" diet. The goal is not to adhere to a strict set of rules or to deprive yourself of foods you enjoy, but rather to develop a healthy and balanced relationship with food that supports your physical, emotional, and spiritual well-being.

Remember, the journey of balancing the chakras is a lifelong one, and there will be times when you may feel more or less grounded and connected to your root chakra. This is a natural part of the human experience, and it's important to approach these fluctuations with compassion and understanding. By nourishing your body with whole, grounding foods and drinks, and by bringing mindfulness and intention to your eating habits, you can support a strong and healthy root chakra. You can cultivate a sense of safety, security, and connection to the earth and your own physical body, even in the midst of life's challenges and uncertainties.

Red Foods, Drinks, Herbs, & Spices

Red apples, beets, tomatoes, pomegranates, strawberries, and raspberries. Root vegetables, including sweet potatoes, carrots, turnips, beets, garlic, parsnips, and onions. Also cacao and chocolate are great for this chakra! Use ginger, turmeric, paprika, cayenne, and horseradish.

Make notes of your favourite combinations or flavours here. Write down a meal that you could make with these ingredients.

A Root Chakra Infusion

• a chunk of fresh ginger, sliced

• half a stick of cinnamon

• a chunk of turmeric root, sliced

• 400ml hot boiled water

Let it all infuse for 5 minutes. You can drink this hot, or let it cool and have it at room temperature, chilled, or over ice, if you prefer. Strain, and pour into your favourite mug or glass, and then make a ritual of drinking it, as below.

An Alternative Root Chakra Drink

Treat yourself to the best hot chocolate you can, or make some hot cocoa, or use ceremonial grade cacao powder to make a luxury drink. Use your favourite cup, and take it to your favourite seat. Bonus points if it's either outside or has a beautiful view of outside! Breathe in the scent. Feel the steam on your face. Sip slowly, savour each mouthful, and let your tongue pick out all the flavours. Feel it travel through your body; follow the sense of heat all the way down. Take the time to drink this mindfully, fully aware of the positive energetic balancing of your root chakra. Feel yourself connected to the earth, filled with the abundance that comes from having enough. Right at this moment, you are safe, warm, and fed. This is safety, and this is abundance

ROOT Day 2: Journal Prompt

Consider the elements of nature associated with grounding, such as earth and roots. How connected do you feel to these elements? What are some memories of nature that feel good to you? Are there specific practices or activities that help you feel more grounded?

ROOT DAY 3: YOGA

Let's explore the transformative power of yoga for the root chakra, or Muladhara. This foundational energy centre is associated with our sense of safety, security, and belonging. When the root chakra is balanced, we feel grounded, stable, and connected to the earth beneath our feet. When this chakra is balanced and open, we feel a strong connection to the earth, a sense of stability in our physical body, and a deep trust in the unfolding of our lives. Yoga offers a powerful set of tools for balancing and activating this chakra. By incorporating specific poses into your practice, you help to release physical and emotional tension, cultivate a sense of grounding and presence, and connect with the inherent stability and support of the earth beneath you.

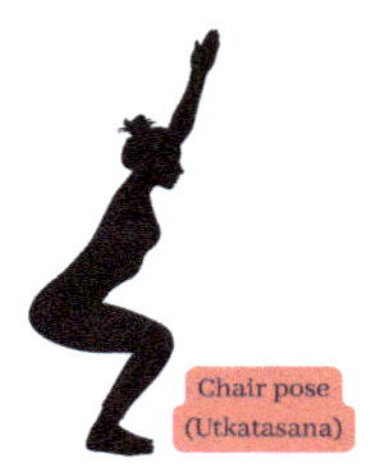

Chair pose
(Utkatasana)

One of the most effective poses for the root chakra is Chair Pose (Utkatasana). This powerful standing posture helps to build strength and stability in the thighs, calfs and feet, while also engaging the core muscles and stimulating the root chakra. Sink your hips back and down, as if sitting in an invisible chair, and create a sense of grounding and connection to the earth, promoting a feeling of safety and security.

Mountain Pose (Tadasana) is another fundamental posture for the root chakra. This simple standing pose helps to establish a strong and stable foundation, and encourages a sense of alignment and balance in the body. As we root down through the feet and lengthen up through the crown of the head, we create a connection between heaven and earth, promoting a feeling of inner strength and stability.

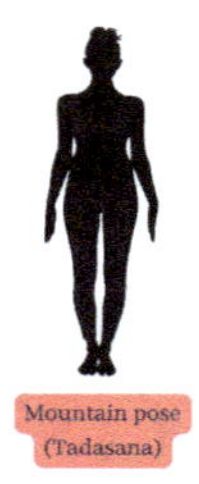

Mountain pose
(Tadasana)

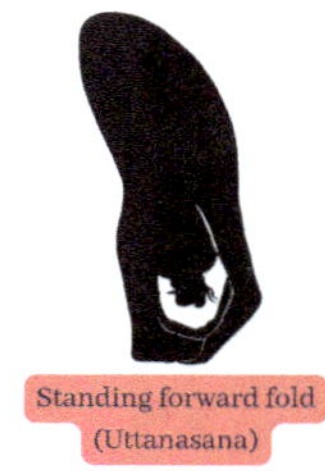

Standing forward fold
(Uttanasana)

Standing Forward Fold (Uttanasana) is a gentle inversion that can help to calm the mind and soothe the nervous system, while also stretching the hamstrings and activating the root chakra. As you fold forward from the hips, allow your head to hang heavy towards the earth. Tilt it from side to side to release any tension in your neck, Absorb a sense of surrender and release, and accept a feeling of letting go and grounding into the present moment.

Knee-to-Chest Pose (Apanasana) is a gentle supine posture that can help to release tension in the lower back and hips, while also promoting a sense of grounding and security. As you lie on your back and hug one or both knees into the chest, you create a sense of compression and support in the root chakra region, promoting a feeling of safety and comfort.

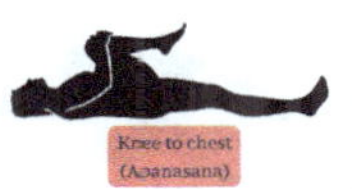

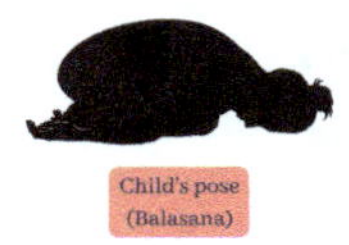

Child's Pose (Balasana) is a restful posture that can help to soothe the mind and calm the nervous system, while also gently stretching the hips, thighs, and lower back. Sit back on your heels and allow your forehead to rest on the ground, or use a cushion or folded blanket to support you if needed. This pose encourages a sense of surrender and release, and a feeling of safety and security in the root chakra.

Garland Pose (Malasana) is a deep squatting posture that can help to open the hips and groin, while also stimulating the root chakra and promoting a sense of grounding and connection to the earth. As you sink the hips down towards the ground and bring your palms together in front of your heart, feel your inherent stability and inner strength. Relax your shoulders and inhabit a feeling of confidence and self-assurance.

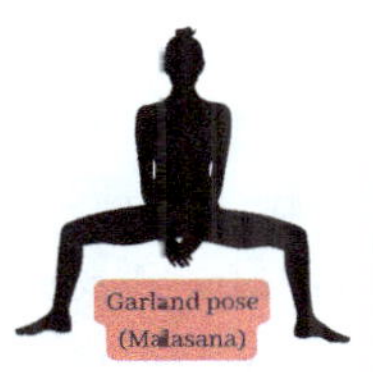

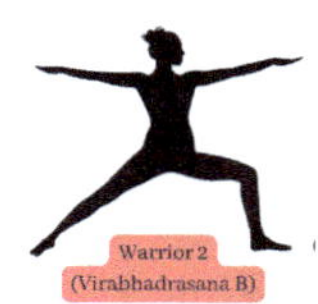

Finally, Warrior II (Virabhadrasana II) is a powerful standing posture that can help to build strength and stability in the legs and core, while also promoting a sense of grounding and inner strength. As you sink into your front knee and extend your arms out to the sides, you create a sense of expansion and vitality in your body. Breathe into this feeling of confidence and personal power.

Incorporating these poses into a regular yoga practice can help to balance and activate your root chakra, supporting you, helping you to develop your own sense of grounding, stability, and inner strength. However, please remember to approach these poses with mindfulness and self-compassion. Listen to your body, breathe gently, and honour your body's unique needs and limitations.In addition to the physical benefits, yoga for the root chakra can also offer profound emotional and spiritual benefits. When you truly connect with the inherent stability and support of the earth, you cultivate a greater sense of trust and faith in the unfolding of your life. You learn to feel safe and secure in your own body, and to develop a deep sense of belonging and connection to the world around you. Ultimately, the journey of awakening, balancing, and nurturing the root chakra is a deeply personal and transformative one. By showing up to your practice with consistency, patience, and an open heart, you'll gradually peel away the layers of fear, insecurity, and disconnection, revealing the inherent stability, strength, and grounding that resides within.

I know this is just day 3, but I encourage you to explore the transformative power of yoga as often as you can – even just a few minutes or a couple of poses a day will do wonders for you. When nurturing your root chakra, trust in the wisdom and support of the earth beneath you. Remember that you are always held and supported, and that by connecting with your own inner foundation, you can create a life of stability, security, and joy.

ROOT Day 3: Journal Prompt

Consider your relationship with movement and exercise. How do you engage with physical activity? Do you feel a sense of joy, challenge, or resistance? How could you find more joy in movement?

ROOT Day 4: EFT

EFT tapping, short for Emotional Freedom Techniques, is a therapeutic technique that combines gentle tapping on specific acupressure points on the body with focused attention on emotional issues. It aims to release emotional blockages and restore balance in the body's energy system. By tapping on these points while acknowledging and addressing emotional concerns, EFT tapping can help alleviate stress, anxiety, and other negative emotions, promoting a sense of emotional well-being.

You begin with a set-up statement, which you repeat three times whilst tapping on the karate chop point. You then repeat an affirmation whilst tapping gently on each tapping point in turn. Don't worry about remembering everything, this page is repeated for each chakra!

Tapping points

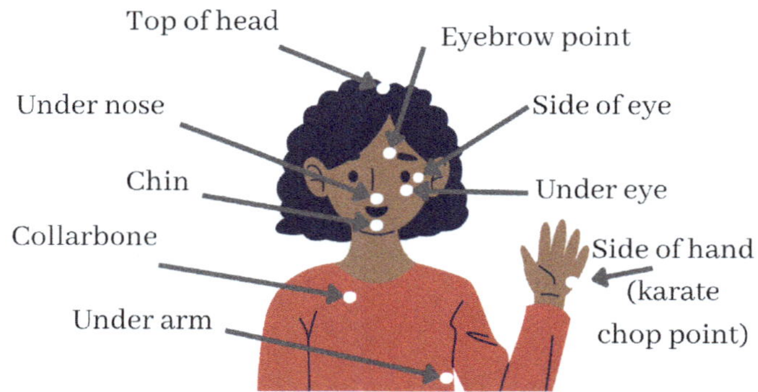

Set up phrase - tap side of hand (karate chop point):
"Even though I am not always grounded, I love and accept myself.

Even though I am not always grounded, I love myself exactly as I am now.

Even though I am not always grounded, I love, honour and accept myself completely."

Eyebrow point: "I am grounded, stable, and secure in all aspects of my life."

Side of eye: "I release fear, and trust in the abundance of the universe."

Under eye: "I am rooted in the present moment, finding strength in the here and now."

Under nose: "I am safe and protected, both physically and emotionally."

Chin: "I embrace change and adapt easily to life's transitions."

Collarbone: "I am connected to the Earth, drawing upon its energy for stability and support."

Under arm: "I deserve to have my basic needs met, and I attract all that I need."

Top of head: "I am a beacon of strength and resilience, standing firm in the face of challenges."

Repeat seven times.

ROOT Day 4: Journal Prompt

Take a moment to tune into your physical body. How do you feel in your body right now? Are there areas of tension? Explore the reasons for these, and what you could do to ease them.

ROOT DAY 5: CRYSTALS & MEDITATION

I f you have one of these crystals, hold it while you follow this meditation. If you don't have one, don't worry. You can hold a picture of one, or simply visualise on in your hands as you meditate. If you'd like me to lead you in this meditation, you can go to my store and download it for free, or find me under Jennifer Jones on the meditation app Insight Timer.

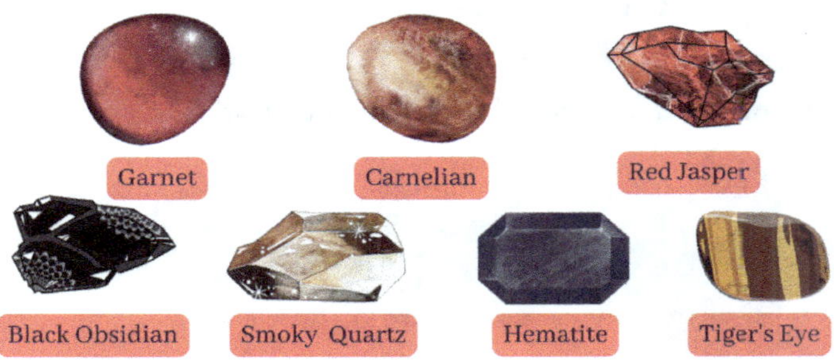

- Find a quiet and comfortable place where you can sit or lie down. Close your eyes and take a few deep breaths to relax.

- Begin by focusing on your breath. Take slow, deep breaths in and out, feeling the sensation of the breath entering and leaving your body. Allow your breath to become slow and steady.

- Direct your attention to the base of your spine, where the root chakra is located. Visualise a vibrant, glowing red light here. Imagine this light growing brighter with each breath, filling your root chakra with warmth and energy.

- As you continue to breathe deeply, bring your awareness to the physical sensations in your body. Notice any areas of tension or discomfort, and imagine the red light from your root chakra gently dissolving and releasing any stagnant energy or negativity stored there.

- As you release tension and negative energy, imagine a sense of stability and grounding spreading throughout your body. Visualise roots growing from your tailbone deep into the earth, anchoring you securely to the ground.

- Stay with this visualisation and continue to breathe deeply for a few more moments, allowing the energy of the root chakra to flow freely and bring a sense of balance and stability to your entire being.

- When you feel ready, slowly bring your awareness back to your surroundings. Gently open your eyes and take a moment to reflect on your experience.

- Note down any thoughts, feelings, observations, or ideas that came to you.

ROOT DAY 5: JOURNAL PROMPT

R eflect on your relationship with your physical body and the material world. How do you feel about your body? How does your attitude towards money, possessions, and material resources impact your sense of stability?

SACRAL

I feel

Sacral Day 1: Physical Activity

The sacral chakra, or Svadhisthana, is associated with our emotions, creativity, and sensuality. When this energy centre is balanced, we feel vibrant, passionate, and able to express ourselves authentically in the world. Engaging in physical activities that help us connect with our bodies and emotions is a powerful way to cultivate balance in the sacral chakra.

One of the most effective ways to tap into the energy of the sacral chakra is through dance. Whether you prefer a structured dance class or simply moving freely to your favourite music at home, allowing your body to flow and express itself can be incredibly liberating and empowering. As you move, focus on the sensations in your body, the rhythm of the music, and the emotions that arise. Let go of self-judgment and allow yourself to be fully present in the moment, embracing the joy and vitality of your own unique expression. You don't need to be a 'good' dancer! A quick boogie in the kitchen is a tonic of its own.

Another physical activity that helps balance the sacral chakra is swimming. Immersing yourself in water is incredibly soothing and nurturing. It helps to release emotional blockages and encourages a sense of flow and ease. As you glide through the water, focus on the sensation of your body being supported and held. Release any tension or stress. You may also find it helpful to visualise the water washing away any stagnant or negative energy, leaving you feeling refreshed and rejuvenated.

Here's an amazing and surprising practice that you may reject out of hand at first – belly dancing! Belly dancing is a wonderful way to connect with your body, sensuality, and creative expression, making it an excellent practice for balancing the sacral chakra. Remember, belly dancing is a celebration of your body and your creative essence, so enjoy the process and let your authentic self shine through. With regular practice, you'll find that belly dancing not only supports the balance of your sacral chakra but also enhances your overall sense of confidence, vitality, and self-expression.

As you explore these various physical activities, remember to approach them with a spirit of curiosity and self-compassion. Rather than striving for perfection or achievement, focus on the journey itself, allowing each moment to unfold with presence and acceptance. Trust that by nurturing your sacral chakra through these practices, you are cultivating a deeper sense of emotional intelligence, creativity, and vitality that will ripple out into all areas of your life.

Choose One of the Following Activities

Freeform Dance

Put on some music that makes you feel alive and inspired, and allow your body to move freely and spontaneously. Let go of any self-consciousness or judgment, and simply focus on the sensations of your body moving through space. As you dance, bring your awareness to your hips and pelvis, imagining the energy of the sacral chakra flowing freely and vibrantly. Allow yourself to express any emotions that arise, whether through movement, sound, or simply being present with the experience.

Swimming

Visit a local pool, lake, or ocean and immerse yourself in the water. As you swim, focus on the sensation of the water flowing around your body, supporting and cradling you. Imagine any stress, tension, or emotional blockages being washed away with each stroke, leaving you feeling cleansed and refreshed. You may also find it helpful to incorporate playful movements, such as floating on your back or doing gentle twists and turns, to promote a sense of flexibility and ease.

Belly Dancing

Take a belly dancing class or practice at home. There are plenty of online instructors with free videos, so if you feel self-conscious you can immerse yourself in this in privacy at home! Having said that, it might also be a fun activity to do with a trusted friend. If you just want to give it a try without connecting to a screen, try this:

Find a comfortable space where you can move freely, and put on music that inspires you to dance. Start by gently swaying your hips from side to side, focusing on the fluid, circular motions of your pelvis. As you become more comfortable, incorporate more complex movements, such as figure eights, shimmies, and undulations. Allow your arms to flow gracefully with your movements, and feel free to add

your own unique flair and style. As you dance, bring your awareness to
your lower abdomen, visualizing a vibrant orange energy glowing and
swirling in your sacral chakra. Embrace the sensations of pleasure, creativity, and emotional flow that arise, letting go of any self-judgment
or inhibition. Let yourself get lost in the music, and focus on the fluid
movements of the hips and pelvis to connect with your sensuality and
creativity.

Sacral Day 1: Journal Prompts

What activities or hobbies bring you joy and ignite your creativity? Reflect on activities that make you feel alive, inspired, and engaged. Explore how these activities can help you tap into your creative energy and cultivate a sense of joy.

Sacral Day 2: Foods, Drinks, Herbs & Spices

Tody we'll enjoy the foods that can support the sacral chakra, Svadhisthana. To support a sense of balance and vitality in the sacral chakra, it's important to focus on foods and drinks that are nourishing, energising, and emotionally satisfying. These foods tend to be rich in natural sugars, healthy fats, and vibrant colours, reflecting the qualities of sweetness, pleasure, and creativity that are associated with this chakra.

One of the key components of a sacral chakra-balancing diet is an emphasis on foods that are naturally sweet and full of flavour. These foods can help to stimulate the senses and promote feelings of pleasure and satisfaction, while also providing a source of quick and easily accessible energy. As well as this, find foods that are rich in Omega 3s, which help to control inflammation and are essential in so many physiological processes. Some specific foods that can be particularly nourishing for the sacral chakra include:

Fruits: Fruits are naturally sweet and hydrating, making them an excellent choice for balancing the sacral chakra. Opt for juicy, colourful fruits like oranges, mangoes, strawberries, and passion fruit, which are rich in vitamins, antioxidants, and other nutrients that support overall health and vitality. These fruits can be enjoyed on their own as a snack, or incorporated into smoothies, salads, and other dishes.

Nuts and seeds: Nuts and seeds are rich in healthy fats, protein, and minerals like zinc and magnesium, which are important for reproductive health and emotional well-being. They are also a great source of energy and can help to promote feelings of satiety and satisfaction. Try incorporating almonds, cashews, pumpkin seeds, and sesame seeds into your diet, either as a snack or as a topping for salads and other dishes.

Whole grains: Whole grains like brown rice, quinoa, and oats are rich in complex carbohydrates, which provide a slow and steady release of energy throughout the day. They are also a good source of fibre, which can help to promote healthy digestion and elimination. When combined with other nourishing foods like vegetables and lean proteins, whole grains can help to create a sense of balance and satisfaction in the body.

Leafy greens: Leafy green vegetables like spinach, kale, and chard are packed with vitamins, minerals, and other nutrients that support overall health and vitality. They are also rich in chlorophyll, which can help to purify the blood and promote a sense of clarity and focus. Try incorporating leafy greens into your diet on a regular basis, either as a salad, a sautéed side dish, or a smoothie ingredient.

Spices: Certain spices can be particularly nourishing for the sacral chakra, thanks to their warming, energising properties. Cinnamon, ginger, and cardamom are all great choices, as they can help to stimulate circulation, boost energy levels, and promote feelings of pleasure and satisfaction. Try incorporating these spices into your cooking, or enjoying them in the form of herbal teas or warm milks.

In addition to these specific foods, it's important to focus on eating a balanced and varied diet that includes plenty of fresh, whole foods. Aim to incorporate a range of colours and textures into your meals, as this can help to stimulate the senses and promote feelings of creativity and vitality.

When it comes to drinks, water is once again a key component of a sacral chakra-balancing diet. In addition to staying hydrated with plain water, you may also want to experiment with infusing your water with fresh fruits, herbs, and spices. This can help to add flavour and nutrients to your water, while also promoting feelings of pleasure and satisfaction.

Other drinks that can be supportive for the sacral chakra include herbal teas, particularly those made with warming spices like ginger and cinnamon, as well as fresh juices and smoothies made with nourishing fruits and vegetables.

As with the root chakra, it's important to approach your sacral chakra-balancing diet with a sense of mindfulness and intention. Use your creativity and passion to create beautiful dishes, even if you don't consider yourself to be a great cook. It's less about making a five-star meal, and more about acknowledging the love you feel for yourself, mindfully nourishing yourself and takign time to consider how the foods you eat will make your body feel. You deserve to be well fed and cared for, and even if all you have time for is beans on toast, give yourself the time to fully enjoy and appreciate it. Take the time to enjoy your meals, savouring the flavours, textures, and aromas of your food. Eat slowly and with gratitude, tuning in to your body's natural hunger and fullness cues.

By nourishing your body with vibrant, flavourful foods and drinks, and by embracing your own unique sense of creativity and sensuality, you can support a healthy and balanced sacral chakra. You can tap into your inner source of joy, passion, and emotional vitality, even in the midst of life's ups and downs.

Orange Foods, Drinks, Herbs, & Spices

Carrots, mango, oranges, orange peppers, peaches, apricots, and sweet potatoes. Salmon, tuna, and oily fish. Nuts and seeds such as flax, almonds, walnuts, and sesame. Coconut, and spices such as cinnamon, liquorice, turmeric with black pepper, and whole roasted cumin seeds. Stay hydrated and drink plenty of water, coconut water, or herbal teas like dandelion or rose hip. Make some notes below about meals you could create using these ingredients.

A Sacral Chakra Infusion

- 10 whole cardamom pods
- 1 teaspoon whole fennel seeds
- ¼ teaspoon unsweetened vanilla powder
- 400ml hot boiled water

Let it all infuse for 5 minutes. You can drink this hot, or let it cool and have it at room temperature, chilled, or over ice, if you prefer. Strain, and pour into your favourite mug or glass, and then make a ritual of drinking it.

An alternative root chakra drink

Coconut, orange & mango smoothie. One orange, some frozen mango, frozen banana, full fat coconut milk and some coconut oil, blended together,

Take the time to really enjoy this drink, fully aware of the positive energetic balancing of your sacral chakra.

Sacral Day 2: Journal Prompts

How do I embrace my sensuality and honour my body? Is it through foods, particular textures of clothes or bedding, through baths, showers, body oils or creams? Is it by moving to music or seeing a piece of art that moves you? Explore your relationship with your body and sensuality. Reflect on ways you can embrace and celebrate your physicality, nurturing a healthy and loving connection with your body.

Sacral Day 3: Yoga

Today's sacral balancing activity will be yoga. as we've discovered, this vibrant energy centre is associated with our creativity, sensuality, and emotional flow. When the sacral chakra is balanced, we feel alive, passionate, and connected to our inner source of joy and pleasure. Yoga offers a beautiful way to tap into this energy of the sacral chakra, inviting us to explore our creative potential and emotional depths. By incorporating specific poses that target this area, we cultivate a sense of fluidity, flexibility, and openness, both in our physical body and our emotional landscape.

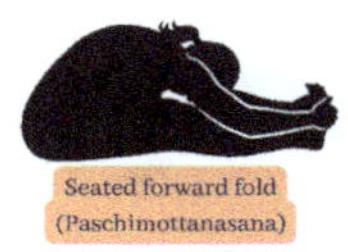
Seated forward fold (Paschimottanasana)

One powerful pose for the sacral chakra is Paschimottanasana, or Seated Forward Bend. As you fold forward, reach for your toes and surrender the weight of your head towards the earth. Don't force the bend, but allow your body to go as far as is comfortable for you. This pose creates a gentle compression in the lower abdomen, stimulating the sacral region, and invites us to let go of any tension or blockages we may be holding onto, allowing our creative energy to flow freely.

Another wonderful pose for the sacral chakra is Prasarita Padottanasana, or Wide-Legged Forward Bend. As you step your feet wide apart and fold forward, you create space in the hips and pelvis, releasing stagnant energy and promoting a sense of openness and receptivity. This pose encourages you to embrace your sensual nature, connecting with the pleasure and joy that is your birthright.

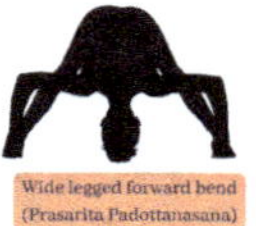

Wide legged forward bend
(Prasarita Padottanasana)

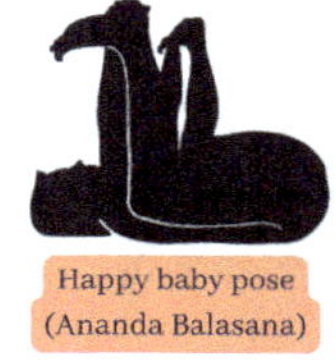

Happy baby pose
(Ananda Balasana)

Ananda Balasana, or Happy Baby Pose, is a playful and nurturing posture that can help to balance the sacral chakra. As you lie on your back and bring your knees towards your chest, grasping your feet with your hands just like a baby discovering their toes, you create a sense of safety and security. Allow yourself to surrender to the present moment. This pose can help to release any emotional blockages or fears, inviting you to connect with your inner child and the joy of simply being.

Setu Bandha Sarvangasana, or Bridge Pose, is a beautiful backbend that can help to open and energise the sacral chakra. Lift your hips towards the sky to create space in the lower back and pelvic region, allowing energy to flow freely. This pose can help to boost your creative potential, inviting you to explore new ideas and possibilities.

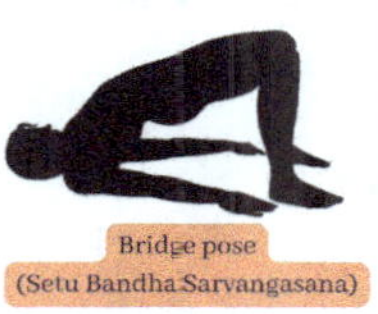
Bridge pose
(Setu Bandha Sarvangasana)

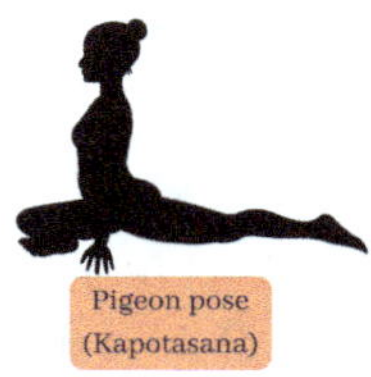
Pigeon pose
(Kapotasana)

Kapotasana, or Pigeon Pose, is a deep hip opener that can be especially beneficial for the sacral chakra. As you fold forward over your front leg, you create a intense stretch in the hip and groin, helping to release any tension or blockages that may be holding you back. This pose can be emotionally as well as physically challenging, inviting you to confront any unresolved issues or fears that may be stored in your hips. By breathing through the discomfort and surrendering to the present moment, you can cultivate a sense of emotional freedom and resilience. Be gentle with yourself, and allow any feelings that arise to flow through you. Don't force anything, physically or emotionally.

Trikonasana, or Triangle Pose, is a standing posture that can help to balance the sacral chakra by creating a sense of spaciousness and expansiveness in the hips and pelvis. As you reach our arm towards the sky, ground down through your

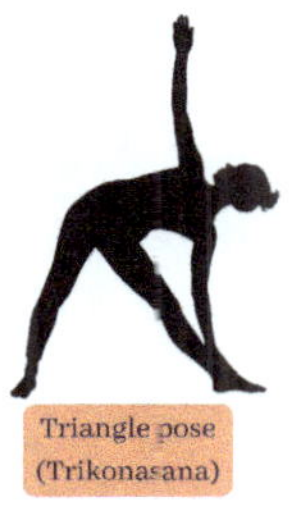
Triangle pose
(Trikonasana)

feet. Invite energy to flow freely through the
sacral region, encouraging a sense of creativity and vitality.

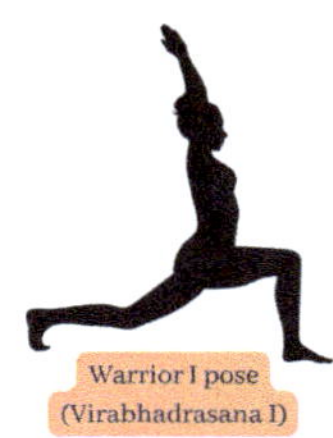

Warrior I pose
(Virabhadrasana I)

Finally, Virabhadrasana I, or Warrior I Pose, is a powerful standing posture that can help to build strength and confidence in the sacral chakra. Sink into your front leg and reach your arms towards the sky. Tap into your inner warrior, cultivating a sense of courage and determination. This pose invites you to embrace your personal power and step forward into the world with boldness and authenticity.

As you explore these sacral chakra yoga poses, remember to listen closely to your body and honour any sensations or emotions that arise. Allow yourself to surrender to the flow of your practice, letting go of any expectations or judgments and simply being present with what is. Trust that by nurturing your sacral chakra through yoga, you are cultivating a deep sense of creativity, sensuality, and emotional freedom that will ripple out into all areas of your life.

sacraL Day 3: JournaL PromPT

What emotions do I need to release or heal? Take time to identify any emotional patterns or wounds that may be holding you back. Explore ways to release and heal these emotions, allowing for greater emotional flow and balance. It may be easier to begin with just one at a time, and let these flow into others if they're called to.

Sacral Day 4: EFT

EFT tapping, short for Emotional Freedom Techniques, is a therapeutic technique that combines gentle tapping on specific acupressure points on the body with focused attention on emotional issues. It aims to release emotional blockages and restore balance in the body's energy system. By tapping on these points while acknowledging and addressing emotional concerns, EFT tapping can help alleviate stress, anxiety, and other negative emotions, promoting a sense of emotional well-being.

You begin with a set-up statement, which you repeat three times whilst tapping on the karate chop point. You then repeat an affirmation whilst tapping gently on each tapping point in turn. Don't worry about remembering everything, this page is repeated for each chakra!

Tapping points

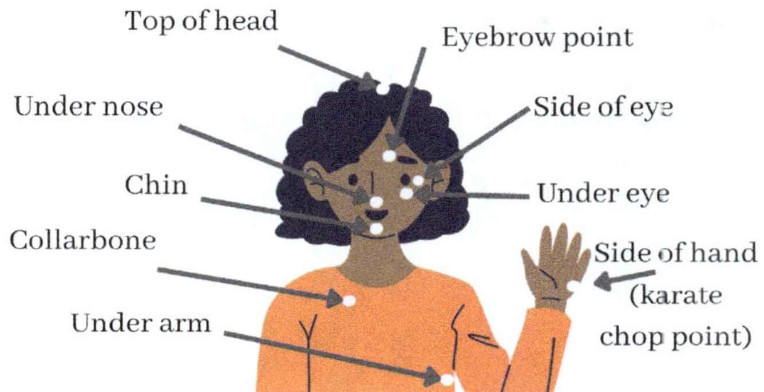

Set up phrase - tap side of hand (karate chop point):

"Even though I don't always express my emotions healthily, I love and accept myself.

Even though I don't always connect to my senses, I love myself exactly as I am now.

Even though I sometimes struggle to be playful and passionate, I love, honour and accept myself completely."

Eyebrow point: "I embrace my creativity and allow it to flow freely in all areas of my life."

Side of eye: "I honour and respect my emotions, allowing them to guide me towards joy and fulfilment."

Under eye: "I embrace my sensuality and find pleasure in the simple joys of life."

Under nose: "I am in touch with my passion and allow it to fuel my desires and goals."

Chin: "I release any guilt or shame surrounding my desires and embrace my authentic self."

Collarbone: "I create healthy and balanced relationships that support my growth and happiness."

Under arm: "I am open to new experiences and allow myself to explore the depths of my desires."

Top of head: "I am connected to my intuition, trusting its guidance in making choices that align with my highest good."

Repeat seven times.

SACRAL DAY 4: JOURNAL PROMPT

Reflect on a time when you felt deeply passionate and alive. Recall a moment in your life when you experienced a strong sense of passion or excitement. What was happening during that time? Did anything particular prompt it? What were the circumstances that enabled it? How can you bring more of that energy into your life now?

Sacral Day : Crystals & Meditation

I f you have one of these crystals, hold it while you follow this meditation. If you don't have one, don't worry. You can hold a picture of one, or simply visualise on in your hands as you meditate. If you'd like me to lead you in this meditation, you can go to my store and download it for free, or find me under Jennifer Jones on the meditation app Insight Timer.

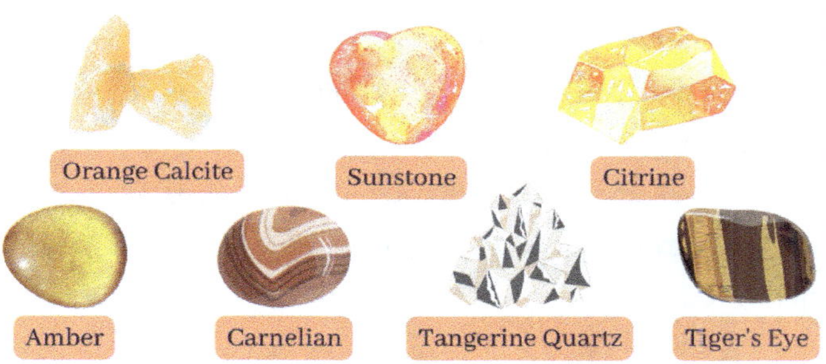

• Find a comfortable and quiet space where you can relax without distractions. Sit or lie down in a comfortable position, closing your eyes, and taking a few deep breaths to centre yourself.

• Visualise a warm, glowing orange light at the area of your lower abdomen, where the sacral chakra is located. Imagine this light expanding and growing brighter with each breath, filling your entire pelvic area with its radiant energy.

• As you continue to breathe deeply, imagine the orange light swirling and spinning in a clockwise direction, clearing any blockages or stagnant energy within the sacral chakra. Feel a sense of warmth and vitality emanating from this energy centre.

• Bring your attention to the qualities associated with the sacral chakra. Visualise yourself engaging in activities that ignite your creativity, such as painting, dancing, or writing. Embrace the pleasure and joy these activities bring to your life.

•Notice what emotions rise up as you visualise this. Notice what you embrace and what you resist, and see how your emotions are connected to these activities. Allow yourself to feel these emotions fully, without judgment or resistance. Acknowledge any emotions that arise and allow them to flow through you, knowing that you have the strength and balance to handle them with grace and compassion.

• Remain in this meditative state for as long as you feel comfortable, soaking in the healing energy of the sacral chakra. When you are ready, take a few deep breaths, gradually bringing your awareness back to the present moment. Gently open your eyes and carry the revitalizing energy of the sacral chakra with you throughout your day.

• Note down any thoughts, feelings, observations, or ideas that came to you.

Sacral Day 5: Journal Prompt

How can I cultivate healthy boundaries in my relationships? Explore your boundaries within relationships—whether personal or professional. Reflect on ways you can establish and maintain healthy boundaries that honour your needs and values.

SOLAR PLEXUS

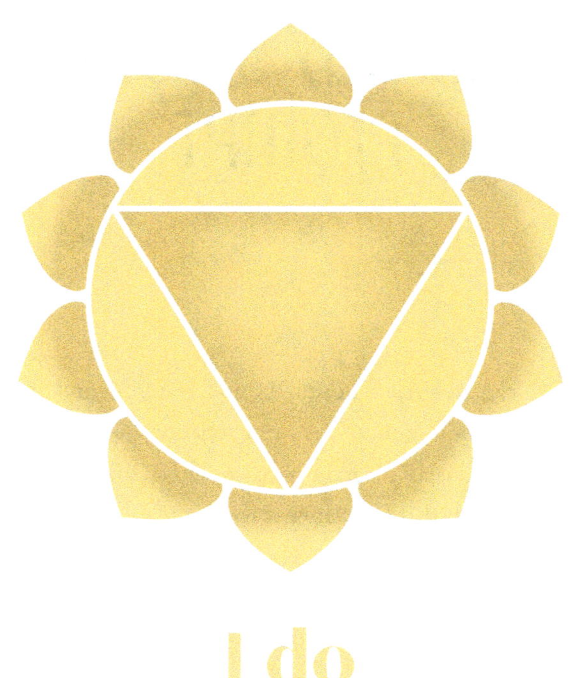

I do

SOLaR PLEXUS DaY 1: PHYSICAL ACTIVITY

The solar plexus chakra, located just above the navel, is associated with our sense of personal power, self-esteem, and self-discipline. When this energy centre is balanced, we feel confident, motivated, and capable of taking action towards our goals and dreams. Engaging in physical activities that challenge us and help us build inner strength is a powerful way to cultivate balance in the solar plexus chakra.

One effective way to boost the energy of the solar plexus chakra is through cardiovascular exercise. Activities such as running, cycling, or skipping can help us build endurance, increase our metabolism, and release endorphins, the body's natural "feel-good" chemicals. As you engage in these activities, focus on the sensations of your body working hard, your heart pumping, and your breath flowing. Embrace the challenge and remind yourself of your own inner strength and resilience. It's okay if it's hard! It's okay if you only exercise for five minutes – or two! The object of the exercise is not to feel defeated and unfit, but to remind yourself how much your body is capable of, and feel proud of yourself for giving it the opportunity to move with energy.

Martial arts, as mentioned in the root chakra section, can also be incredibly beneficial for the solar plexus chakra. The discipline, focus, and self-control required in these practices can help us develop a deep sense of inner strength and personal power. As you move through the techniques and stances, visualise yourself overcoming obstacles and challenges with grace and determination. Remember that your true power lies not in physical strength alone, but in the strength of your spirit and the clarity of your intention.

If you aren't able to do such physically challenging exercises, don't worry! Another great way of using your body to nurture your solar plexus chakra is through the use of affirmations and positive self-talk. Affirmations are short, powerful statements that help to reprogram our subconscious mind and cultivate a more positive, empowered mindset. By repeating affirmations specifically tailored to the solar plexus chakra, we can strengthen our sense of self-worth, confidence, and personal power.

As you explore these physical activities, remember to approach them with mindfulness and self-awareness. Notice any thoughts or emotions that arise, and allow yourself to process them with compassion and understanding. Celebrate your victories and learn from your setbacks, knowing that each experience is an opportunity for growth and self-discovery. Trust that by nurturing your solar plexus chakra through these practices, you are cultivating a deep sense of personal power, self-esteem, and resilience that will support you in all areas of your life.

Choose One of the Following Activities

High-Intensity Interval Training (HIIT)

Find a safe space to exercise, and begin with a few minutes of gentle stretching to warm up your body. Then, engage in a series of high-intensity exercises, such as burpees, mountain climbers, or jumping jacks, for 30 seconds each, followed by 30 seconds of rest. Repeat this cycle for 10-15 minutes, pushing yourself to your personal edge while still listening to your body's needs. As you move through the exercises, focus on your breath and the sensations of strength and vitality coursing through your body.

Affirmations

Find a quiet, comfortable space where you can sit or stand with good posture. Place one hand on your solar plexus area, just above your navel, and take a few deep, centring breaths. As you inhale, imagine a bright, golden light growing and expanding in your solar plexus chakra. As you exhale, envision any self-doubt, fear, or negative energy releasing from your body. Now, begin repeating affirmations that resonate with you, such as:

"I am confident, capable, and worthy of success."
"I trust my inner wisdom and make decisions with ease and clarity."
"I embrace my personal power and use it for the highest good."
"I am resilient, strong, and able to overcome any challenge."

Speak these affirmations out loud, with conviction and enthusiasm. Allow yourself to fully embrace the positive energy and intentions behind each statement. You can also write your affirmations down in a journal, or create visual reminders by posting them around your living space. If you make affirmations a regular part of your daily routine, you'll begin to notice a shift in your thoughts, emotions, and overall energy. Your solar plexus chakra will become more balanced and vibrant, supporting you in all areas of your life. Remember, the power of affirmations lies in consistent practice and genuine belief in the statements you are making. Approach this practice with patience, self-compassion, and an open heart, trusting in the transformative potential of your own words and intentions.

Kickboxing

Find a local kickboxing class or follow along with an online video tutorial. Begin with a warm-up that includes stretches and basic punches and kicks. As you move through the combinations, focus on your breath and the power behind each movement. Visualise yourself breaking through any obstacles or limitations, both inner and outer. Remember that your true strength lies in your ability to stay focused, disciplined, and committed to your goals. End your session with a few minutes of stretching and deep breathing, allowing yourself to integrate the lessons and energy of the practice.

SOLar PLexus Day 1: JOUrnaL PrOmPT

What does personal power mean to me? Reflect on your understanding of personal power and how it manifests in your life. Explore how you can cultivate a sense of personal empowerment and assertiveness.

Solar Plexus Day 2: Foods, Drinks, Herbs, & Spices

Today is all about supportive nutrition for the solar plexus chakra, or Manipura, the seat of our personal power, self-esteem, and inner fire. When the solar plexus chakra is balanced, we feel confident, capable, and in control of our lives. We have a strong sense of purpose and direction, and we are able to navigate challenges and setbacks with resilience and grace. We're able to set healthy boundaries, stand up for ourselves and our beliefs, and take responsibility for our choices and actions.

To support this sense of empowerment and vitality in the solar plexus chakra, it's important to focus on foods and drinks that are energising, strengthening, and supportive of our digestive fire. These foods tend to be warming, slightly spicy, and rich in complex carbohydrates and lean proteins, providing a sustained source of energy and nourishment.

Some specific foods that can be particularly supportive of the solar plexus chakra include:

Yellow foods: In chakra theory, the colour yellow is associated with the solar plexus chakra, and eating foods that are naturally yellow in colour can help to stimulate and balance this energy centre. Good options include yellow bell peppers, squash, corn, and bananas. These foods are also rich in vitamins and minerals that support overall health and vitality.

Lean proteins: Protein is essential for building and repairing tissues in the body, and it can also help to promote feelings of strength and empowerment. Good sources of lean protein for the solar plexus chakra include chicken, turkey, fish, tofu, and legumes like lentils and chickpeas. These foods provide a sustained source of energy and can help to keep us feeling full and satisfied throughout the day.

Complex Carbohydrates: Complex carbohydrates like whole grains, sweet potatoes, and root vegetables provide a slow and steady release of energy, helping to fuel our physical and mental activities. They are also rich in fibre, which supports healthy digestion and elimination. When combined with lean proteins and healthy fats, complex carbohydrates can help to create a sense of balance and vitality in the body.

Spices: Certain spices are particularly nourishing for the solar plexus chakra, thanks to their warming, energising properties. Turmeric, ginger, cumin, and coriander are all great choices, as they can help to stimulate digestion, boost immunity, and promote feelings of inner fire and motivation. Try incorporating these spices into your cooking, or enjoying them in the form of herbal teas or supplements.

Fermented foods: Fermented foods like yogurt, kefir, sauerkraut, and kimchi are rich in beneficial bacteria that support healthy digestion and immune function. They can also help to promote feelings of strength and resilience in the face of stress and challenges. Try incorporating small amounts of fermented foods into your diet on a regular basis, either as a condiment or a side dish.

In addition to these specific foods, it's important to focus on eating a balanced and nourishing diet that supports your overall health and well-being. Aim to incorporate a variety of fresh whole foods into your meals, and limit your intake of processed, sugary, and fried foods, which can be draining and depleting to the solar plexus chakra. When it comes to drinks, water is, of course, a key component of a solar plexus chakra-balancing diet. Aim to drink plenty of pure, clean water throughout the day, and consider infusing your water with energising and detoxifying ingredients like lemon, ginger, or mint.

Other drinks that can be supportive of the solar plexus chakra include herbal teas, particularly those made with warming and stimulating herbs like ginger, turmeric, and dandelion root. These teas can help to promote healthy digestion, boost energy levels, and support the body's natural detoxification processes.

As with the other chakras, it's important to approach your solar plexus chakra-balancing diet with mindfulness and self-compassion. Listen to your body's needs and desires, and honour your own unique preferences and dietary requirements. Eat slowly and with intention, savouring the flavours and textures of your food, and taking the time to express gratitude for the nourishment you are receiving.

Yellow Foods, Drinks, Herbs, & Spices

Bananas, pineapple, corn, lemons, and yellow curry. Also, include complex carbohydrates like oats, brown rice, spelt, rye, beans, vegetables, and sprouted grains. Try adding milk thistle, ginger, turmeric, dandelion, lemon balm, or chamomile to your dishes, or to make tea.

Write down any favourites from this list and any meal ideas you could prepare and enjoy.

A Solar Plexus Chakra Infusion

• 1 thick slice of organic orange with peel

• 1 cinnamon stick

• 8 whole cloves

• 400ml hot boiled water

Let it all infuse for 5 minutes. You can drink this hot, or let it cool and have it at room temperature, chilled, or over ice, if you prefer. Strain, and pour into your favourite mug or glass, and then make a ritual of drinking it.

An alternative solar plexus chakra dish

Make a warming, energising chickpea yellow curry, full of turmeric, black pepper and ginger. Serve with a fennel and dandelion leaf salad. Let yourself enjoy the preparation of this meal, and serve yourself with love, fully aware of the positive energetic balancing of your solar plexus chakra.

SOLar PLexus Day 2: Journal Prompt

Today, explore your strengths, talents, and achievements. Reflect on the areas where you may be holding onto self-doubt or fear of failure. What are you good at? What are you proud of yourself for? And where do you self-sabotage or undermine yourself? Bonus points if you can do this next bit! Text a trusted friend and ask them this question: "What am I good at, that you think I take for granted?" Take their words, write them down, and believe them!

Solar Plexus Day 3: Yoga

Today's solar plexus balancing activity uses yoga. This chakra is associated with our sense of personal power, self-esteem, and self-confidence. When this chakra is balanced and open, we feel a strong sense of purpose, motivation, and inner strength. We are able to take action towards our goals, assert ourselves in the world, and maintain healthy boundaries in our relationships. The yoga poses today will help to release physical and emotional blockages, cultivate a sense of inner fire and determination, and connect with our authentic power and potential.

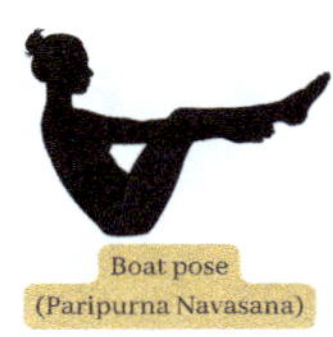

Boat pose
(Paripurna Navasana)

One of the most effective poses for the solar plexus chakra is Boat Pose (Navasana). This challenging core-strengthening posture helps to build heat and fire in the belly, while also cultivating a sense of inner strength and resilience. As you balance on your sitting bones and extend your legs and arms forward, you engage the deep muscles of the abdomen, stimulating the digestive fire and promoting a sense of confidence and personal power.

Cat/Cow Pose (Marjaryasana/Bitilasana) is another beneficial posture for the solar plexus chakra. This gentle flow helps to release tension in the spine and stimulate the flow of energy through the central channel of the body. Inhale and arch the back, creating space for the breath to expand fully into the belly, activating the solar

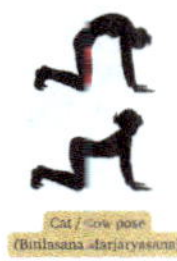

Cat / Cow pose
(Bitilasana Marjaryasana)

plexus and promoting a sense of vitality and aliveness. Then exhale and round the back, to engage the core muscles, and build strength and stability in the abdominal region.

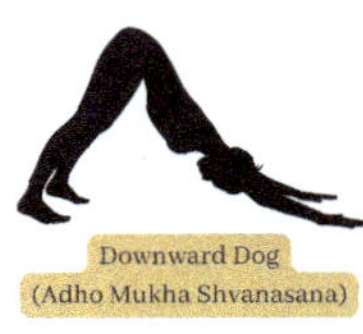

Downward Dog
(Adho Mukha Shvanasana)

Downward Facing Dog (Adho Mukha Svanasana) is a foundational yoga posture that offers numerous benefits for the solar plexus chakra. This pose helps to lengthen the spine, stretch the hamstrings, and activate the core muscles. Press your hands and feet into the earth and lift your hips towards the sky to create a sense of grounding and stability, while also allowing the energy to flow freely through the body. This pose can help to alleviate digestive issues, boost metabolism, and promote a sense of inner strength and vitality. As well as this, the inversion increases blood flow to our brain, heart, and lungs.

Plank Pose (Phalakasana) is another powerful posture for the solar plexus chakra. This pose requires significant core strength and stability, as we hold the body in a straight line, engaging the deep muscles of the abdomen and the arms. By building heat and fire in the belly, Plank Pose can help to boost confidence, increase willpower, and 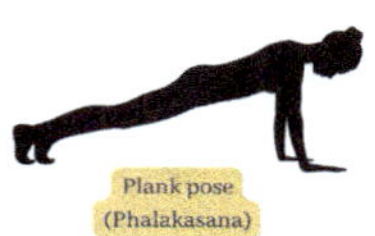 promote a sense of personal power and determination. It contributes to having a super strong core physically, which can only help support your emotional and spiritual core when done mindfully.

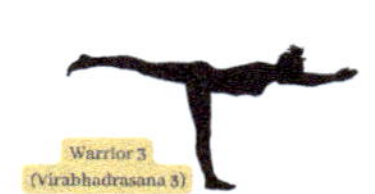 Warrior III (Virabhadrasana III) is a challenging balance posture that can help to activate this chakra. This pose requires focus, concentration, and inner strength, as you stand on one leg and extend the other leg back behind you, reaching your arms forward. By engaging the deep muscles of the core and legs, Warrior III helps to build stability and power in the solar plexus region, promoting a sense of confidence and self-assurance.

Camel Pose (Ustrasana) is a deep backbend that helps to open the chest, stretch the front body, and activate the solar plexus chakra. This pose requires a sense of surrender and trust, as we kneel on the ground and reach the hands back towards the heels. By creating a sense of expansion and freedom in the abdominal region,

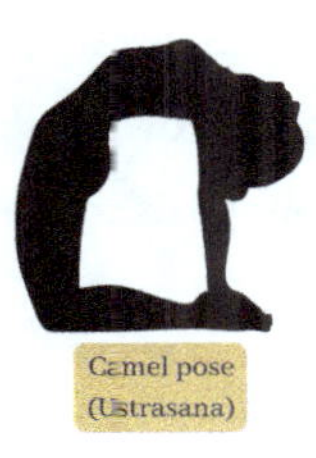
Camel pose (Ustrasana)

Camel Pose helps to release physical and emotional blockages, encouraging a sense of openness and vulnerability.

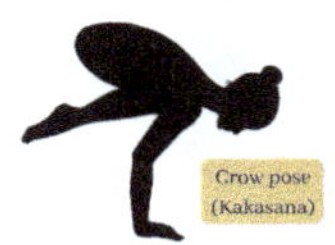
Crow pose (Kakasana)

Finally, Crow Pose (Bakasana) is an advanced arm balance that requires significant core strength, focus, and inner trust. Don't feel that you have to engage with this pose; there are plenty of other suggestions that will be equally beneficial for this chakra. This pose helps to build confidence, increase willpower, and promote a sense of personal power and determination. As you place your hands on the ground and lift your feet off the earth, you engage the deep muscles of the core and the arms, creating a sense of stability and strength in the solar plexus region.

Incorporating these poses into a regular yoga practice can help to balance and activate the solar plexus chakra, enabling a sense of confidence, personal power, and inner strength to grow. However, it is important to approach these poses with care and mindfulness, honouring your body's limitations and listening to any sensations or feelings that arise.

In addition to the physical benefits, yoga for the solar plexus chakra can also offer profound emotional and spiritual benefits. By connecting with our inner fire and personal power, you cultivate a greater sense of self-awareness, self-acceptance, and self-love. You learn to trust in your own abilities, set healthy boundaries, and take action towards your goals and dreams.

Solar Plexus Day 3: Journal Prompt

What fears or self-limiting beliefs hold me back from stepping into my power? Identify those self-doubts that may be inhibiting your personal power. Reflect on their origins. Are they from home life, school, friendships? Where in your body do you feel them? Consider ways you could overcome these limitations. How can you physically move this discomfort out of your body?

Solar Plexus Day 4: EFT

EFT tapping, short for Emotional Freedom Techniques, is a therapeutic technique that combines gentle tapping on specific acupressure points on the body with focused attention on emotional issues. It aims to release emotional blockages and restore balance in the body's energy system. By tapping on these points while acknowledging and addressing emotional concerns, EFT tapping can help alleviate stress, anxiety, and other negative emotions, promoting a sense of emotional well-being.

You begin with a set-up statement, which you repeat three times whilst tapping on the karate chop point. You then repeat an affirmation whilst tapping gently on each tapping point in turn. Don't worry about remembering everything, this page is repeated for each chakra!

Tapping points

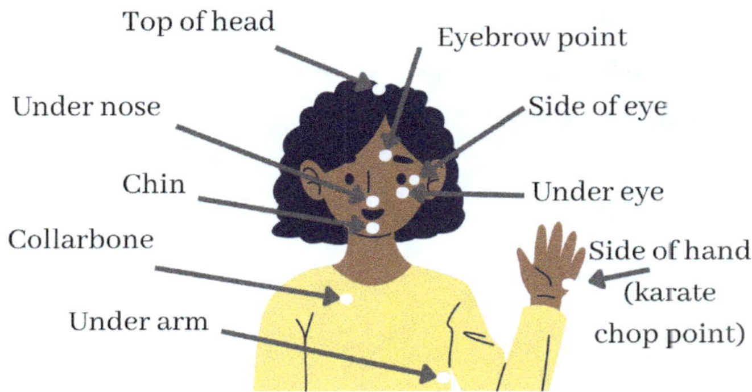

Set up phrase - tap side of hand (karate chop point):

"Even though I don't always feel confident, I love and accept myself.

Even though I don't always feel empowered, I love myself exactly as I am now.

Even though I can be overly critical of myself and others, I love, honour and accept myself completely."

Eyebrow point: "I am confident and empowered, radiating my unique power and strength."

Side of eye: "I trust in my ability to make decisions with clarity and conviction."

Under eye: "I am worthy of success, abundance, and personal fulfilment."

Under nose: "I embrace my personal power and use it responsibly for the highest good of myself and others."

Chin: "I am in control of my life and create positive change with purpose and intention."

Collarbone: "I release self-doubt and step into my authentic self with confidence and courage."

Under arm: "I deserve of love, respect, and recognition for my accomplishments and contributions."

Top of head: "I align my actions with my personal values, creating harmony and balance in all aspects of my life."

Repeat seven times.

SOLAR PLEXUS DAY 4: JOURNAL PROMPT

Recall an instance when you made a choice with a strong sense of clarity and conviction. What were the circumstances that enabled you to feel confident? What factors contributed to those moments? How can you tap into that decision-making power more consistently?

Solar Plexus Day 5: Crystals & Meditation

If you have one of these crystals, hold it while you follow this meditation. If you don't have one, don't worry. You can hold a picture of one, or simply visualise on in your hands as you meditate. If you'd like me to lead you in this meditation, you can go to my store and download it for free, or find me under Jennifer Jones on the meditation app Insight Timer.

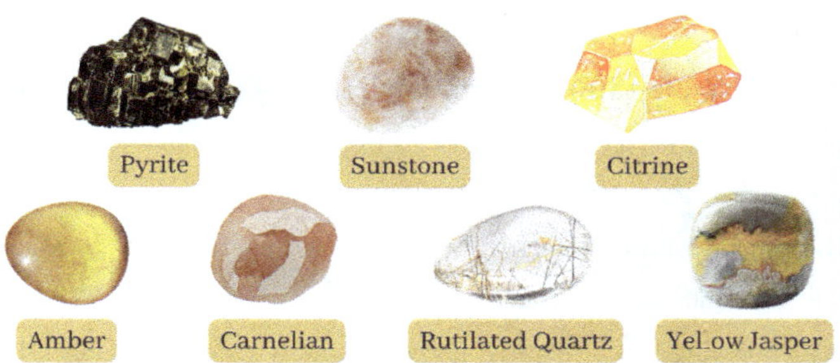

• Find a quiet and comfortable space where you can sit or lie down without interruptions. Close your eyes and take a few deep breaths, allowing your body and mind to relax.

• Visualise a radiant yellow light at the area of your upper abdomen, where the solar plexus chakra is located. Envision this light growing brighter with each breath, filling your entire abdominal region with its warm and vibrant energy.

• As you continue to breathe deeply, imagine the yellow light expanding and spinning in a clockwise direction, clearing away any blockages or stagnant energy and filling you with power and confidence.

• Feel this personal power and inner strength emanate through every area of your body, through your torso, your limbs, your fingers. and toes, your head, face and eyes. Visualise yourself standing tall and assertive, radiating confidence and self- assurance in all aspects of your life.

• Imagine your self-esteem as a bubble around you, shining. alight on all your unique qualities, talents, and accomplishments. Affirm your self-worth whilst envisioning this golden light glowing from you, lighting up the positive impact you have on the world around you. Acknowledge and embrace this sense of self- acceptance and self-love, and notice how it feels to hold this sensation of acceptance in your body.

• Remain in this meditative state, basking in the healing golden glow. of your own power, for as long as you desire. When you're ready,, take a few deep breaths, gradually bringing your awareness back to the present moment. Gently open your eyes, and carry your sense of empowerment and confidence with you into your day, and beyond, remembering that you. can come back to it whenever you need to.

• Note down any thoughts, feelings, observations, or ideas that came to you.

SOLAr PLEXUS DaY 5: JOUrnaL PrompT

How can I cultivate self-discipline and motivation to pursue my goals? Are you generally quite self-motivated, or do you procrastinate until things are desperate? Does it depend on the circumstances? Reflect on which times you were filled with enthusiasm to fulfil a task, and consider strategies that can help you stay focused, committed, and driven in pursuing what truly matters to you.

HEART

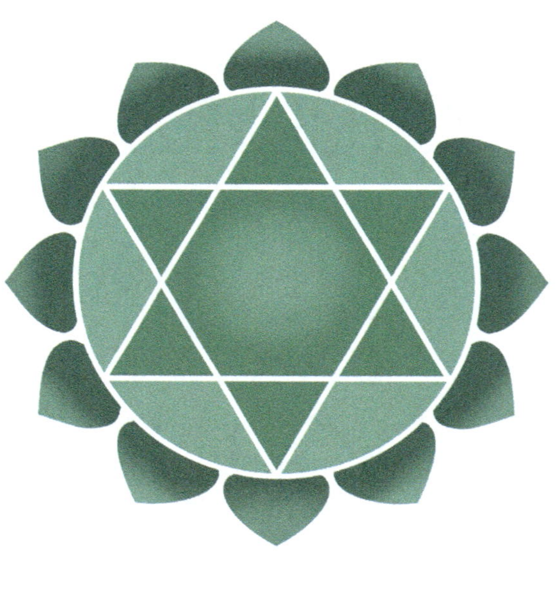

I love

Heart Day 1: Physical Activity

The heart chakra, located in the centre of the chest, is associated with love, compassion, and emotional healing. When this energy centre is balanced, we feel open, connected, and able to give and receive love freely. Engaging in physical activities that promote a sense of joy, connection, and emotional well-being can help cultivate balance in the heart chakra.

One powerful way to nurture the heart chakra is through activities that involve being in nature. Spending time outdoors, surrounded by the beauty and tranquility of the natural world, can help us feel more grounded, peaceful, and connected to all living things. Whether you prefer a gentle wander through the woods, a scenic bike ride, or simply sitting in a park and admiring the trees and flowers, allowing yourself to be present and absorb the healing energy of nature can be incredibly nourishing for the heart chakra.

Another physical activity that can help balance the heart chakra is partner dancing. Engaging in dances such as salsa, tango, or ballroom dancing requires trust, communication, and emotional connection with another person. It doesn't have to be a formal dance, though. Connecting with your partner and dancing in your own way will have exactly the same effect. As you move together in rhythm, focus on the sensations of physical touch and the exchange of energy between you and your partner. Allow yourself to be fully present at the moment, releasing any fears or inhibitions and opening your heart to the joy and intimacy of the dance.

Volunteering and engaging in acts of service is also incredibly beneficial for the heart chakra. When we give our time and energy to help others, we cultivate a deep sense of compassion, empathy, and interconnectedness. Whether you choose to volunteer at a local animal shelter, participate in a community clean-up project, or simply perform random acts of kindness for strangers, focusing on the needs of others can help shift our perspective and open our hearts to the beauty and resilience of the human spirit.

As you explore these physical activities, remember to approach them with a spirit of openness and self-reflection. Notice any emotions or sensations that arise, and allow yourself to process them with gentleness and understanding. Remember that true healing and growth often involve facing our vulnerabilities and learning to love and accept ourselves fully. Trust that by nurturing your heart chakra through these practices, you are cultivating a deep sense of emotional intelligence, compassion, and resilience that will support you in all your relationships and endeavours.

> Choose One of the Following Activities

Nature Walk with Mindful Observation

Go for a walk in a natural setting, such as a park, forest, or beach. As you walk, bring your attention to the beauty and wonder of the natural world around you. If you can't walk, find somewhere beautiful to sit, or sit somewhere and consciously notice any beauty that you see! Notice the colours, textures, and patterns of the plants and animals you encounter. Take deep breaths and allow yourself to be fully present at the moment, absorbing the peaceful energy of your surroundings. If you feel called to do so, whilst walking, find a quiet spot to sit and observe the natural world more deeply, allowing yourself to feel a sense of connection and unity with all living things.

Partner Dance Class

Find a local dance studio or community centre that offers partner dance classes, such as salsa, tango, or ballroom dancing. Attend a class with an open mind and a willingness to learn and connect with others. As you move through the steps and techniques, focus on the sensations of physical touch and the exchange of energy between you and your partner. Remember that partner dancing is a collaborative experience, requiring trust, communication, and mutual respect. Alternatively, make a playlist of your favourite songs, and find somebody to dance with that you love. Observe the exchange of energy that occurs when you are totally connected with the body and movements of another person.

Volunteer at a Local Community Organisation or Offer Donations

Research local community organisations that align with your values and interests, such as a food bank, animal shelter, or environmental conservation group. Sign up for a volunteer shift and approach the experience with a spirit of service and compassion. As you engage in the tasks and activities of the organisation, focus on the positive impact you are making in the lives of others and the larger community. Allow yourself to feel a sense of connection and purpose, knowing that your efforts are contributing to the greater good. If you can't donate your time, consider what abundance you have in your home that you could offer. Could you declutter an area (also supporting the root chakra!), clear out a closet or add some items from your supermarket shop into the local food donation bank? Remember that acts of service not only benefit others but also help to open and heal our own hearts in profound ways.

Heart Day 1: Journal Prompt

How do I express love and compassion towards myself? Reflect on how you talk to yourself when times are tough. Explore self-care practices, self-acceptance, and ways to nurture a loving relationship with yourself.

Heart Day 2: Foods, Drinks, Herbs, & Spices

Today, we feed our heart chakra, Anahata, the centre of love, compassion, and emotional healing. We're going to care for this gentle, powerful energy centre and strengthen our ability to give and receive love, to connect with others from a place of empathy and understanding, and to experience the deep sense of inner peace and contentment that comes from living in alignment with our true nature.

When the heart chakra is balanced, we feel a profound sense of love and acceptance for ourselves and others. We're able to form deep and meaningful relationships, to communicate our needs and desires with clarity and kindness, and to approach life's challenges with an open and compassionate heart. We can forgive and release past hurts and traumas, and cultivate a sense of gratitude and appreciation for the blessings in our lives.

To support this sense of love and emotional balance in the heart chakra, it's important to focus on foods and drinks that are nourishing, comforting, and energetically uplifting. These foods tend to be rich in healthy fats, antioxidants, and other nutrients that support cardiovascular health and emotional well-being, while also providing a sense of warmth and satisfaction.

Some specific foods that can be particularly supportive of the heart chakra include:

Leafy greens: Leafy green vegetables like spinach, kale, and Swiss chard are packed with vitamins, minerals, and antioxidants that support overall health and vitality. They are also rich in magnesium, a mineral that is essential for heart health and emotional balance. Try incorporating leafy greens into your diet on a regular basis, either as a salad, a sautéed side dish, or a smoothie ingredient.

Berries: Berries like strawberries, raspberries, and blueberries are rich in antioxidants and other nutrients that support cardiovascular health and emotional well-being. They are also naturally sweet and satisfying, making them a great choice for those who crave something sweet but want to avoid processed sugars. Try enjoying berries on their own as a snack, or adding them to yogurt, oatmeal, or smoothies.

Avocados: Avocados are rich in healthy monounsaturated fats, which have been shown to support heart health and reduce inflammation in the body. They are also a good source of fibre, potassium, and other nutrients that support overall health and well-being. Try incorporating avocados into your diet as a spread on toast, a topping for salads, or a creamy addition to smoothies.

Cacao: Raw cacao is a powerful superfood that is rich in antioxidants, magnesium, and other nutrients that support emotional balance and heart health. It is also a natural mood-booster, thanks to its high levels of feel-good compounds like theobromine and phenylethylamine. Try incorporating raw cacao into your diet in the form of cacao nibs, cacao powder, or dark chocolate (aim for varieties with at least 70% cacao content).

Green tea: Green tea is a gentle and uplifting beverage that is rich in antioxidants and other nutrients that support heart health and emotional well-being. It is also a natural source of L-theanine, an amino acid that promotes relaxation and reduces stress and anxiety. Try enjoying a cup of green tea in the morning or afternoon as a soothing and energising pick-me-up.

Besides these specific foods and drinks, it's important to focus on eating a balanced and nourishing diet that supports your overall health and well-being. Aim to incorporate a variety of fresh, whole foods into your meals, and limit your intake of processed, sugary, and inflammatory foods, which can be taxing on the heart and emotions. For drinks, water is once again a key component of a heart chakra-balancing diet. Aim to drink plenty of pure, clean water throughout the day, and consider infusing your water with heart-supportive ingredients like rose petals, hibiscus, or lemon balm.

Other beverages that can be supportive for the heart chakra include herbal teas, particularly those made with soothing and uplifting herbs like chamomile, lavender, and hawthorn berry. These teas can help to promote relaxation, reduce stress and anxiety, and support overall emotional well-being. As with the other chakras, it's important to approach your heart chakra-balancing diet with compassion and self-love. Honour your body's unique needs and desires, and listen to the wisdom of your own heart. Eat with mindfulness and gratitude, savouring the flavours and textures of your food, and taking the time to appreciate the love and care that went into preparing it. Always remember that true healing and balance in the heart chakra comes from within, and no external substance or experience can replace the power of self-love and self-acceptance. By nourishing your body with wholesome, heart-supportive foods and drinks, and by cultivating a deep sense of love and compassion for yourself and others, you can support a healthy and balanced heart chakra, and experience the profound sense of peace and connection that comes from living with an open heart.

Green Foods, Drinks, Herbs, & Spices

Raw foods, and leafy and cruciferous vegetables. Kale, broccoli, spinach, chard, dandelion greens, parsley, celery, cucumber, courgette, matcha, green tea, avocado, lime, mint, peas, kiwi, peas, spirulina, green apples, brussels sprouts, bok choy, cabbages and leeks. Have a nourishing bowl of miso soup, drink fresh green juices, or make yourself a green smoothie.

Note down any foods from this list that you like and could nourish yourself with. Write a recipe or meal idea for your heart chakra supporting days.

A Heart Chakra Infusion

- 1 tablespoon dried rosebuds
- 400ml hot boiled water

Let all infuse for 5 minutes. You can drink this hot, or let it cool and have it at room temperature, chilled, or over ice, if you prefer. Strain, and pour into your favourite mug or glass, and then make a ritual of drinking it.

An alternative heart chakra dish

Have a hearty bowl of pea and broccoli soup, with a side of kale and brussels sprouts salad with quinoa and roasted tofu. Use your favourite bowl, and take it to your favourite seat. Bonus points if it's either outside or you can see the outside! Breathe in the scent. Feel the steam on your face. Sip slowly, savour each mouthful, and let your tongue pick out all the flavours. Feel it travel through your body; follow the sense of heat all the way down. Take the time to enjoy this mindfully, fully aware of the positive energetic balancing of your heart chakra. Feel gratitude for loving yourself enough to make nourishing food.

Heart Day 2: Journal Prompt

Reflect on a moment when you experienced deep connections and love with others. Recall instances in your life when you felt a profound connection and love towards others. What qualities or experiences contributed to those moments? How can you cultivate more of those connections in your life?

Heart Day 3: Yoga

It's lovely to balance the heart chakra with these yoga poses. Hopefully by now, about half way our journey of balancing the chakras, you are really feeling the benefit of chakra-centred yoga. Today we are of course taking care of the heart chakra, also known as Anahata. It's the fourth energy centre and is associated with our ability to give and receive love, compassion, and empathy. When this chakra is balanced and open, we feel a deep sense of connection and unconditional love for ourselves and others, and are able to express ourselves with authenticity and vulnerability. Yoga will help to release physical and emotional tension, cultivate a sense of openness and receptivity, and connect with your inner source of love and compassion.

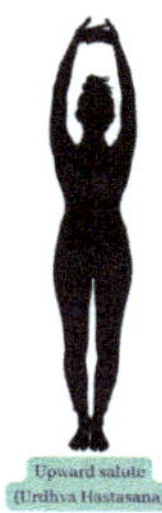

Upward salute
(Urdhva Hastasana)

One of the most effective poses for the heart chakra is also one of the simplest: Upward Salute (Urdhva Hastasana). This simple standing posture opens the chest and shoulders, while also encouraging a sense of upliftment and joy. As you reach your arms towards the sky and gaze upward, you create a sense of expansion and openness in the heart centre, promoting a feeling of connection and gratitude.

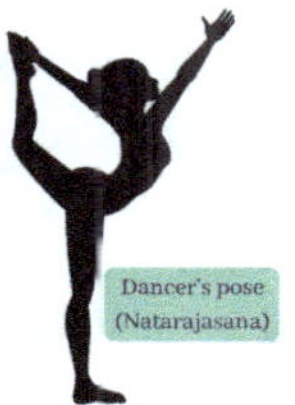

Dancer's pose
(Natarajasana)

Dancer's Pose (Natarajasana) is another powerful posture for the heart chakra. It requires a steady leg and is best if you're comfortable balancing (one good trick is to fix your gaze on a single point ahead of you). This beautiful balancing pose opens the chest and shoulders, while also giving you a sense of grace and self-expression. As you reach back and grasp the foot with one hand, extending your other arm forward, you create a sense of expansion and freedom in the heart centre, promoting a feeling of love and acceptance for ourselves and others.

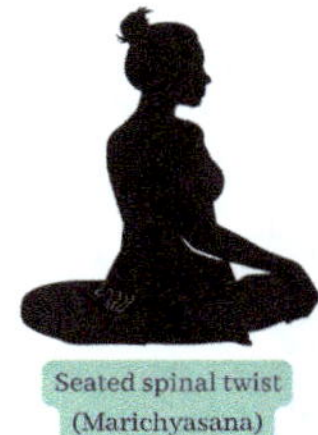

Seated spinal twist
(Marichyasana)

Seated Spinal Twist (Ardha Matsyendrasana) is a gentle twisting posture that can help to release tension in the spine and shoulders, while also encouraging detoxification and renewal in the body. As you twist to one side, allowing the opposite shoulder to relax and the gaze to soften, you open your heart and your receptivity. Twist to either side, brething gently, and inhaling a feeling of letting go and forgiveness.

Bound Ankle Pose (Baddha Konasana) is a gentle hip-opening posture that helps to release emotional tension and promotes a sense of inner peace and tranquility. As you sit with the soles of the feet together and your knees wide, you feel openness and receptivity in the heart centre, promoting a feeling of self-love and acceptance.

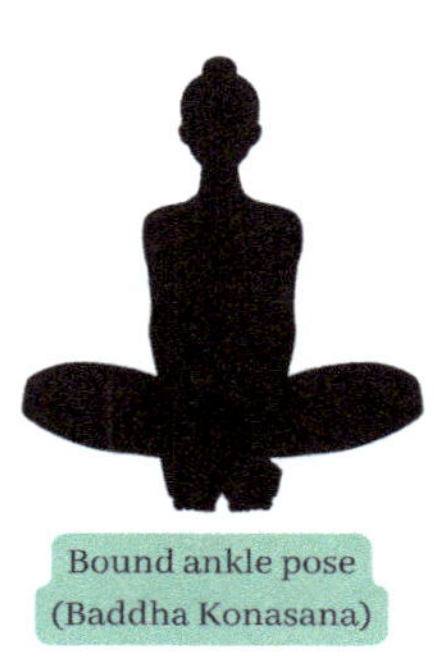

Bound ankle pose
(Baddha Konasana)

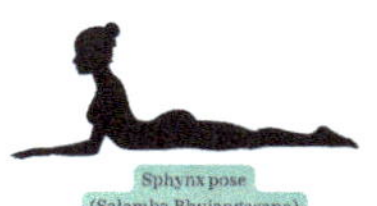

Sphynx pose
(Salamba Bhujangasana)

Sphinx Pose (Salamba Bhujangasana) is a gentle backbend that can help to open the chest and shoulders, while also allowing a sense of emotional healing and self-discovery. Lie on your stomach and lift your chest off the ground, supporting yourself with the forearms. Breathe here, creating a sense of expansion and freedom in the heart centre, allowing a feeling of courage and vulnerability to settle within you.

Bow Pose (Dhanurasana) is a deeper back-bend that can help to open the chest and shoulders, while also encouraging emotional release and transformation. Lie on your stomach and lift your chest and legs off the ground, grasping both ankles with your hands. This pose allows

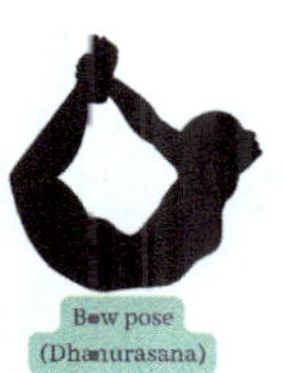

expansion and freedom in the heart chakra, encouraging a feeling of letting go and surrendering to the present moment.

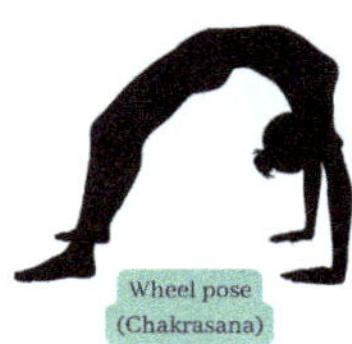

Finally, Wheel Pose (Urdhva Dhanurasana) is a powerful backbend that can help to open the chest and shoulders, while also promoting a sense of emotional healing and self-empowerment. Be sure you are comfortable before attmepting this as it can feel challenging. If you're at all unsure, choose another pose to practise instead – yoga should be enjoyable, not scary! Lift your hips off the ground and press your hands and feet into the earth. This pose creates a sense of expansion and vitality in the heart chakra, promoting a feeling of courage, strength, and resilience.

Incorporating these poses into a regular yoga practice can help to balance and activate the heart chakra, promoting a sense of love, compassion, and emotional healing in our lives. However, it is important to approach these poses with mindfulness and self-compassion, honouring the body's unique needs and limitations. In addition to the physical benefits, yoga for the heart chakra can also offer profound emotional and spiritual benefits. By connecting with our inner source of love and compassion, we can cultivate a greater sense of self-awareness, self-acceptance, and self-love. We can learn to express ourselves with authenticity and vulnerability, and to cultivate deep and meaningful relationships with others.

Heart Day 3: Journal Prompt

What emotional wounds or past hurts need healing in order to open my heart fully? Identify any emotional wounds or past hurts that may be blocking your ability to fully open your heart. Reflect on ways to heal and release these wounds, allowing for greater emotional freedom and love.

Heart Day 4: EFT

EFT tapping, short for Emotional Freedom Techniques, is a therapeutic technique that combines gentle tapping on specific acupressure points on the body with focused attention on emotional issues. It aims to release emotional blockages and restore balance in the body's energy system. By tapping on these points while acknowledging and addressing emotional concerns, EFT tapping can help alleviate stress, anxiety, and other negative emotions, promoting a sense of emotional well-being.

You begin with a set-up statement, which you repeat three times whilst tapping on the karate chop point. You then repeat an affirmation whilst tapping gently on each tapping point in turn. Don't worry about remembering everything, this page is repeated for each chakra!

Tapping points

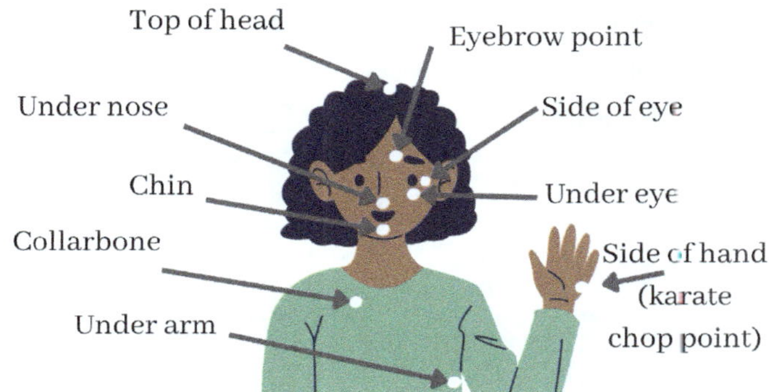

Set up phrase - tap side of hand (karate chop point):

"Even though I feel lonely and unloved, I love and accept myself.

Even though I judge myself and others, I love myself exactly as I am now.

Even though I don't always take good care of myself, I love, honour and accept myself completely."

Eyebrow point: "I am open to giving and receiving love unconditionally."

Side of eye: "My heart is a source of compassion and kindness towards myself and others."

Under eye: "I forgive myself and others, releasing any past hurts and embracing healing."

Under nose: "I choose love over fear and allow love to guide my actions and decisions."

Chin: "I am connected to the universal love that flows through all beings."

Collarbone: "I live in harmony and balance, nurturing meaningful connections and relationships."

Under arm: "I deserve of love and joy, and I attract loving and supportive relationships into my life."

Top of head: "I send love and healing energy to all parts of myself, embracing self-love and self-acceptance."

Repeat seven times.

Heart Day 5: Crystals & Meditation

I f you have one of these crystals, hold it while you follow this meditation. If you don't have one, don't worry. You can hold a picture of one, or simply visualise on in your hands as you meditate. If you'd like me to lead you in this meditation, you can go to my store and download it for free, or find me under Jennifer Jones on the meditation app Insight Timer.

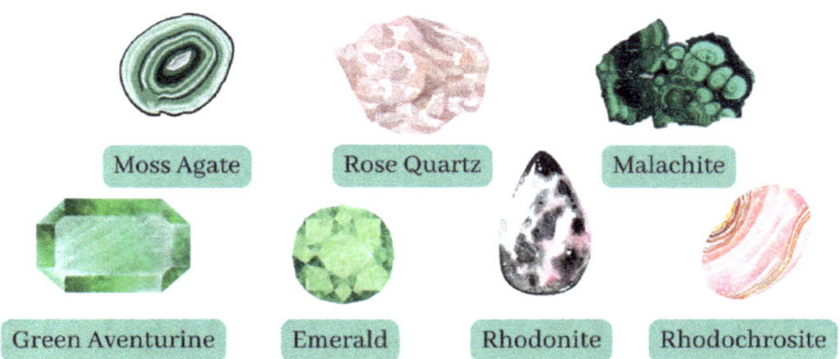

• Find a quiet and comfortable space where you can sit or lie down without distractions. Close your eyes and take a few deep breaths, allowing yourself to relax and let go of any tension.

• Visualise a radiant green light at the centre of your chest, where the heart chakra is located. Imagine this light growing brighter with each breath, expanding to fill your entire chest area with gentle and soothing warmth.

• As you continue to breathe deeply, visualise the green light expanding outward, creating a sphere of loving energy around your heart. Feel this sphere expanding and encompassing your entire body, bathing you in healing and compassionate energy.

• Bring your attention to the qualities associated with the heart chakra. Feel the sphere around you fill with love, compassion, and forgiveness. Visualise yourself surrounded by love, both receiving and radiating it to others. Embrace a sense of deep compassion and understanding for yourself and those around you.

• Allow any emotions that arise to be acknowledged and embraced with compassion. Imagine the green light gently washing away any emotional pain or hurt, replacing it with a profound sense of healing and peace.

• Remain in this meditative state, basking in the healing energy of the heart chakra, for as long as you want. When you're ready, take a few deep breaths, gradually bringing your awareness back to the present moment. Gently open your eyes, carrying the loving and compassionate energy of the heart chakra with you into your interactions and experiences for the rest of your day.

• Note down any thoughts, feelings, observations, or ideas that came to you.

Heart Day 5: Journal Prompt

Create a gratitude journal specifically for expressing gratitude from your heart. Begin to write down all the things that you are grateful for, whether big or small, obvious or obscure. Write what it is about those things that makes you feel grateful, being as specific as possible to really tap into how lucky you feel. You can choose a certain number of things, if you want, set a timer and fill seven minutes with gratitude, or begin an open-ended list that you add to regularly, until you have a seemingly endless collection of blessings.

THROAT

I speak

THROAT DAY 1: PHYSICAL ACTIVITY

The throat chakra, located at the base of the throat, is associated with communication, self-expression, and speaking one's truth. When this energy centre is balanced, we feel confident in our ability to express ourselves authentically and listen deeply to others. Engaging in physical activities that promote clear communication, creative expression, and active listening can help cultivate balance in the throat chakra.

One powerful way to nurture the throat chakra is through singing or chanting. Whether you prefer to sing along to your favourite songs in the car, join a local choir, or simply hum to yourself in the shower, the act of using your voice to create sound can be incredibly freeing and empowering. As you sing or chant, focus on the vibrations of your voice resonating in your throat and throughout your body. It doesn't matter if you think you are good at singing or not! This is simply about using your voice, especially if you shy away from sharing it. Allow yourself to express your emotions fully, releasing any tension or blockages and letting your authentic self shine through

Another physical activity that can help balance the throat chakra is journaling or creative writing. The act of putting pen to paper and allowing our thoughts and feelings to flow freely is a powerful form of self-expression and emotional release. Whether you choose to write in a structured format, such as morning pages or a gratitude journal, or simply allow yourself to free-write without judgment, the process of translating your inner world into words can help you gain clarity, insight, and a deeper understanding of yourself and others.

Engaging in activities that require active listening and clear communication, such as public speaking or participating in a debate club, can also be beneficial for the throat chakra. These experiences challenge us to articulate our thoughts and ideas clearly and effectively while also practicing the skill of listening deeply to others' perspectives. As you engage in these activities, focus on speaking from a place of authenticity and integrity, while also remaining open and receptive to feedback and differing viewpoints. Remember that true communication is a two-way street, requiring both honest self-expression and compassionate understanding.

As you explore these physical activities, remember to approach them with patience, curiosity, and self-compassion. Notice any fears or insecurities that arise around self-expression and allow yourself to gently push past them, trusting in your own unique voice and perspective. Celebrate your progress and learning opportunities, knowing that each experience is a chance to grow and evolve. Trust that by nurturing your throat chakra through these practices, you are cultivating a deep sense of authenticity, creativity, and connection that will support you in all your communications and relationships.

Choose One of the Following Activities

Karaoke Night or Singing Out Loud

Gather some friends or family members and plan a karaoke night, either at home or at a local pub. Choose songs that resonate with you emotionally and allow yourself to fully embody the lyrics and melody as you sing. Let go of any self-consciousness or fear of judgment, and focus on the joy and freedom of expressing yourself through music. As you sing, imagine your voice resonating with the energy of your throat chakra, releasing any blockages and filling you with a sense of confidence and authenticity. If you really can't bring yourself to do karaoke – it's not for everyone! – commit to singing somewhere on your own. Maybe in the shower, in the kitchen, or in the car! Put on your favourite songs and let yourself sing as freely as a beloved child might.

Morning Pages

Set aside 15-20 minutes each morning to engage in a free-writing practice known as "morning pages." The idea is to fill three pages of a notebook with stream-of-consciousness writing, without worrying about grammar, spelling, or content. Simply let your thoughts and feelings flow onto the page without judgment or censorship. This practice can help you clear your mind, process emotions, and tap into your inner wisdom and creativity. As you write, focus on the sensation of the pen moving across the page and the words flowing from your heart and mind.

Join a Public Speaking Club

Are you brave when it comes to public speaking, or does the very idea fill you with terror?! Is today the day to face your fear? Research local public speaking organisations, such as Toastmasters, and attend a meeting as a guest. It's a great first step. Observe how the members practice their communication skills and provide feedback and support to one another. If you feel inspired, consider joining the club and participating in the various speaking exercises and opportunities. As you engage in these activities, focus on expressing yourself clearly and authentically, while also practicing active listening and openness to feedback. Remember that public speaking is a skill that can be developed with practice and dedication, and that each experience is an opportunity to grow and learn.

THROAT DAY 1: JOURNAL PROMPT

How do I express my authentic voice and communicate my truth? Reflect on how you express yourself through communication. Explore moments when you felt truly heard and understood. How can you cultivate a more authentic and expressive voice, allowing your truth to be heard? Can you take a pause between thinking and responding, so that you allow your thoughts to be measured? Or is it better when you remove the inner critic and let your thoughts flow freely?

THroaT Day 2: FOODS, DrinKS, HerBS & SPiceS

Let's enjoy some throat chakra nourishing foods and drinks today. The throat chakra, or Vishuddha, is the centre of communication, self-expression, and truth. It's associated with our ability to speak our truth, to express ourselves authentically and creatively, and to communicate with clarity and integrity. When the throat chakra is balanced, we feel a deep sense of ease and flow in our communication. We are able to express ourselves freely and confidently, without fear of judgement or rejection. We listen deeply and empathetically to others, and engage in meaningful and honest dialogue. We are also able to tap into our own inner truth and creativity, and to express ourselves through various forms of art, music, and self-expression.

To support this sense of clear and authentic communication in the throat chakra, it's important to focus on foods and drinks that are nourishing, soothing, and energetically balancing. These foods tend to be rich in vitamins, minerals, and other nutrients that support the health of the throat, voice, and thyroid gland, while also promoting a sense of emotional and spiritual harmony.

Some specific foods that are particularly supportive for the throat chakra include:

Fruits: Fruits like apples, pears, and plums are naturally sweet and hydrating, making them a great choice for soothing and nourishing the throat. They are also rich in vitamins and antioxidants that support overall health and immunity. Try enjoying these fruits on their own as a snack, or incorporating them into smoothies, salads, or baked goods.

Soups: Warm, nourishing soups can be incredibly soothing and supportive of the throat chakra, especially when made with ingredients like ginger, garlic, and turmeric, which have natural anti-inflammatory and immune-boosting properties. Try making a simple vegetable or bone broth soup, or experimenting with different recipes that feature these throat-supportive ingredients.

Herbal Teas: Certain herbal teas can be particularly beneficial for the throat chakra, thanks to their ability to soothe and nourish the throat and voice. Good options include slippery elm tea, which has a naturally mucilaginous quality that can help to coat and protect the throat, as well as licorice root tea, which has a sweet and soothing flavour. Other supportive herbs include marshmallow root, fennel, and chamomile.

Raw Honey: Raw honey has natural antibacterial and anti-inflammatory properties that can help to soothe and protect the throat. It is also a natural source of enzymes, antioxidants, and other nutrients that support overall health and immunity. Try adding a spoonful of raw honey to your tea or warm water, or using it as a natural sweetener in your cooking and baking.

Water: Staying properly hydrated is essential for the health and function of the throat chakra, as well as for overall physical and emotional well-being. Aim to drink plenty of pure, clean water throughout the day, and consider adding a slice of lemon or a sprig of fresh mint for an extra boost of flavour and nutrients.

In addition to these specific foods and drinks, it's important to focus on eating a balanced and nourishing diet that supports your overall health and well-being. Aim to incorporate a variety of fresh, whole foods into your meals, with an emphasis on fruits, vegetables, whole grains, and lean proteins. Limit your intake of processed, sugary, and artificial foods, which can be dehydrating and irritating to the throat and voice. While supporting the throat chakra through diet and nutrition, it's also important to pay attention to how you eat and drink. Take the time to sit down and enjoy your meals in a relaxed and mindful way, chewing your food thoroughly and savouring each bite. Avoid eating on the go or while distracted by technology or other activities, as this can lead to mindless overeating and digestive discomfort.

It's also important to be mindful of any foods or drinks that may be irritating or challenging for your unique throat and voice. Some people may find that certain foods, such as dairy, gluten, or spicy foods, can be irritating to the throat and voice, while others may have no issues with these foods. Listen to your own body and pay attention to any signs of discomfort or irritation, and adjust your diet accordingly.

Blue Foods, Drinks, Herbs, & Spices

Fill your plate with things that are blue in colour, and, because it's important to be hydrated, choose foods with a high water content: Blueberries and blackberries, cantaloupe, honey dew and watermelons, cucumber and celery. Drink fresh water, coconut water, herbal teas, raw honey, and lemon. Fruit that grows on trees such as apples, pears, figs and plums. Foods good for your thyroid such as nori, sea kelp and samphire.

Choose those foods that appeal to you from the list, and make a note of which ones you like and could make a meal, drink, or snack from.

A Throat Chakra Infusion

- 2 sprigs of fresh mint
- 2 sprigs of dried sage
- 1 slice of organic lemon with peel
- 1 tablespoon raw honey
- 400ml hot boiled water

Let all infuse for 5 minutes. You can drink this hot, or let it cool and have it at room temperature, chilled, or over ice, if you prefer. Strain, and pour into your favourite mug or glass, and then make a ritual of drinking it.

An alternative throat chakra drink

Blue Smoothie: Blend raspberries, banana, blueberries, blue spirulina, honey and hemp seeds with water, ice, or your choice of milk. Give yourself the time to enjoy this and sip slowly, mindfully opening your throat chakra and allowing your wisdom to flow freely through your voice.

THROAT DAY 2: JOURNAL PROMPT

What fears or self-doubts hinder my self-expression? Identify any fears or self-doubts that may be inhibiting your ability to express yourself fully. Reflect on their origins and consider ways to overcome these limitations. When do you feel self-conscious in communication, and how could you alleviate this?

THROAT DAY 3: YOGA

The throat chakra, also known as Vishuddha, responds well to yoga, just like all the other chakras! As we move up the body, it's easy to forget that the chakras associate with more spiritual or ethereal qualities are still very much connected to the energy of our physical bodies. This chakra is, of course, associated with our ability to communicate and express ourselves with authenticity, clarity, and truth. When this chakra is balanced and open, we feel a strong sense of self-expression, creativity, and connection to our inner voice and purpose. Yoga helps to release physical and emotional tension, cultivates a sense of openness and clarity, and connects us with our inner source of wisdom and truth.

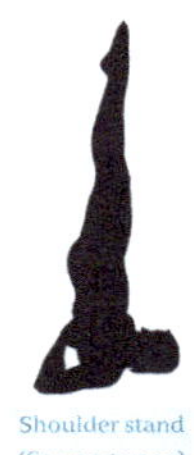

Shoulder stand
(Sarvangasana)

One of the most effective poses for the throat chakra is Shoulder Stand (Sarvangasana). You may need the support of a wall behind you! This inverted posture helps to stimulate the thyroid gland, which is closely associated with the throat chakra and plays a key role in regulating metabolism and energy levels in the body. As you lift the legs and hips overhead and support the body with your shoulders and arms, you create a sense of balance and alignment in the throat chakra, promoting a feeling of clarity and self-expression.

Child's Pose (Balasana) is one of my favourites. It's a gentle resting posture that can help to release tension in the neck and shoulders, while also promoting a sense of introspection and self-reflection. As you sit back on the heels and allow your forehead to rest on the ground (or

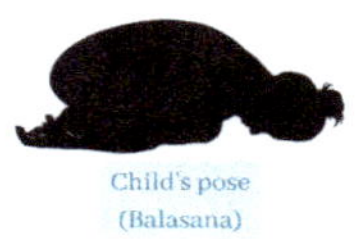

Child's pose
(Balasana)

a cushion, if you need extra support), you create a sense of surrender and receptivity in the throat centre, encouraging a feeling of inner peace and clarity.

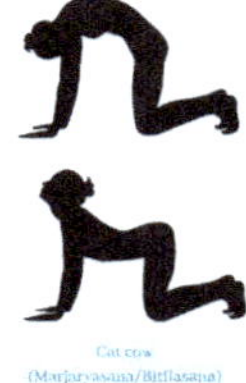

Cat cow
(Marjaryasana/Bitilasana)

Cat-Cow Pose (Marjaryasana-Bitilasana) is another multi-purpose pose. It's gentle flow releases tension in the spine and neck, while also supporting a sense of flexibility and adaptability in the body and mind. As you move between spinal flexion and extension, coordinating your movement with the breath, you create a sense of openness and flu-idity in the throat centre, promoting a feeling of self-expression and creativity.

Bridge Pose (Setu Bandha Sarvangasana) is the gentle backbend that opens the chest and shoul-ders, while also stimulating the thyroid gland and promoting a sense of energy and vitality in the throat chakra. As you lift your hips off the ground and clasp your hands beneath the body,

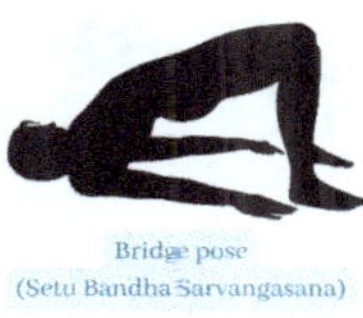

Bridge pose
(Setu Bandha Sarvangasana)

you create a sense of expansion and freedom in the throat chakra, promoting self-expression and communication.

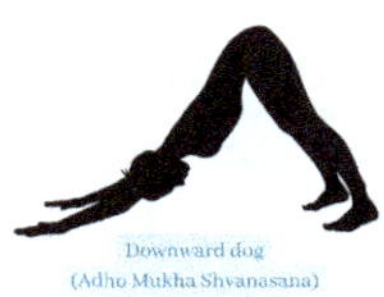

Downward dog
(Adho Mukha Shvanasana)

Downward-Facing Dog Pose (Adho Mukha Svanasana) stretches the spine, shoulders, and hamstrings, giving you a sense of grounding and stability in the body and mind. Press your hands and feet into the earth and lift your hips towards the sky, creating a sense of length and space in the throat centre, encouraging clarity and self-expression.

Plow Pose (Halasana) is a deep forward bend that can help to stretch the spine and shoulders, while also stimulating the thyroid gland and pro-moting a sense of introspection and self-reflec-tion. Be sure you feel comfortable to approach this pose; if not, choose another. It can feel quite

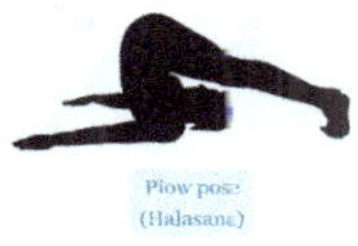

Plow pose
(Halasana)

intense! As you lift your legs overhead and allow your toes to touch the ground behind the head, you feel a sense of surrender and receptivity in the throat centre, allowing a feeling of inner wisdom and intuition.

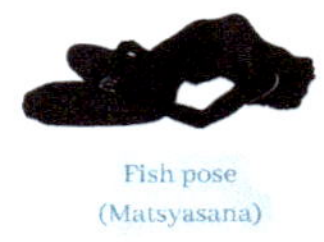

Fish pose
(Matsyasana)

Finally, Fish Pose (Matsyasana) is a gentle backbend that can help to open the chest and throat, while also encouraging emotional release and self-expression. As you lie on your back and lift your chest off the ground, supporting yourself with your elbows and forearms, you create expansion and freedom in the throat centre, allowing a feeling of authenticity and truth.

Incorporating these poses into a regular yoga practice can help to balance and activate the throat chakra, encouraging a sense of self-expression, creativity, and connection to our inner voice and purpose. However, it is important to approach these poses with mindfulness and self-compassion, honouring the body's unique needs and limitations. In addition to the physical benefits, yoga for the throat chakra can also offer profound emotional and spiritual benefits. By connecting with our inner source of wisdom and truth, we can cultivate a greater sense of self-awareness, self-acceptance, and self-expression. We can learn to communicate with authenticity and clarity, and to speak our truth with courage and conviction.

THROAT DAY 3: JOURNAL PROMPT

Reflect on a time when your words had a positive impact on someone. What were the circumstances? Can you remember what exactly it was that you said, or was the important thing either the *way* that you spoke, or simply the fact that you spoke? How did it feel to have that impact? How can you continue to use your voice for positive change?

THROAT DAY 4: EFT

EFT tapping, short for Emotional Freedom Techniques, is a therapeutic technique that combines gentle tapping on specific acupressure points on the body with focused attention on emotional issues. It aims to release emotional blockages and restore balance in the body's energy system. By tapping on these points while acknowledging and addressing emotional concerns, EFT tapping can help alleviate stress, anxiety, and other negative emotions, promoting a sense of emotional well-being.

You begin with a set-up statement, which you repeat three times whilst tapping on the karate chop point. You then repeat an affirmation whilst tapping gently on each tapping point in turn. Don't worry about remembering everything, this page is repeated for each chakra!

Tapping points

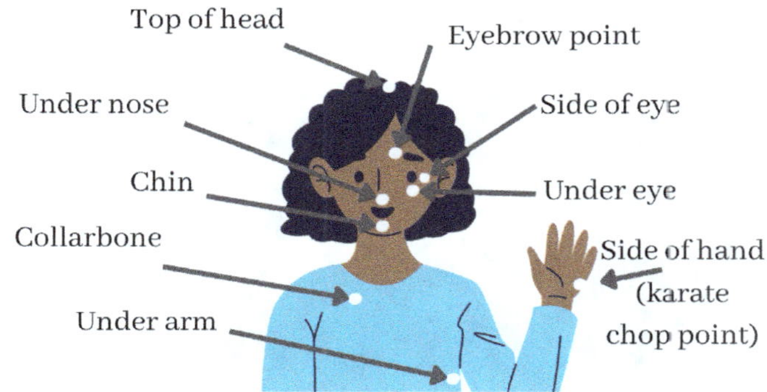

Set up phrase - tap side of hand (karate chop point):

"Even though I don't always express myself clearly, I love and accept myself.

Even though I don't trust my own voice, I love myself exactly as I am now.

Even though I am afraid to speak my truth, I love, honour and accept myself completely."

Eyebrow point: "I express myself confidently and authentically."

Side of eye: "My voice is powerful and worthy of being heard."

Under eye: "I communicate my thoughts and feelings with clarity and ease."

Under nose: "I speak my truth with integrity and courage."

Chin: "I embrace my unique creativity and share it with the world."

Collarbone: "I listen attentively and communicate with empathy and understanding."

Under arm: "I trust in my ability to communicate effectively and positively influence others."

Top of head: "I honour my words and use them to uplift, inspire, and create positive change."

Repeat seven times.

THROAT DAY 4: JOURNAL PROMPT

Explore the role of silence and stillness in communication. Are you comfortable sitting in silence with someone, or do you feel the need to fill the silence with words? How can you cultivate moments of silence and presence, allowing for deeper connection and understanding? What could you practise to help you feel more comfortable, if that is something you feel would be beneficial?

THROAT DAY 5: CRYSTALS & MEDITATION

If you have one of these crystals, hold it while you follow this meditation. If you don't have one, don't worry. You can hold a picture of one, or simply visualise on in your hands as you meditate. If you'd like me to lead you in this meditation, you can go to my store and download it for free, or find me under Jennifer Jones on the meditation app Insight Timer.

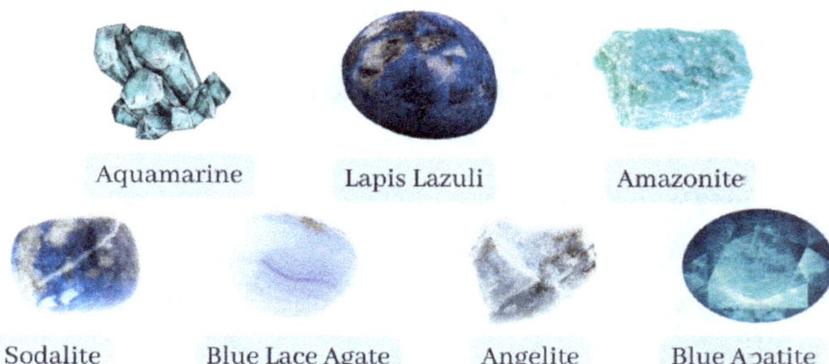

• Find a quiet and comfortable space where you can peacefully sit or lie down.. Close your eyes and take a few deep breaths, allowing your body and mind to relax.

• Visualise a bright blue light at the base of your throat, where the throat chakra is located. Imagine this blue light swirling and spinning in a clockwise direction, clearing any blockages or stagnant energy within the throat chakra.

• Feel this light expand with each breath, filling your entire throat area with its vibrant and calming energy as you inhale, surrounding you and filling your energy field as you exhale.

• Continue breathing deeply and slowly. Feel a sense of clarity and openness emanating from this energy centre.

• Visualise yourself speaking your thoughts and feelings with confidence, clarity and kindness. See your authenticity travelling out on a beam of blue light, directly from your throat. Imagine your communication flowing as effortlessly as a stream down a mountain.

• See the space around you as a safe, healing space of compassionate, active listening. Meaningful and authentic communication flows to and from you. You feel safe speaking and listening. Absorb the blue light into every cell of your body.

• Basking in this healing energy for as long as you want. When you're ready, wiggle your fingers and toes and take a few deep breaths, gradually bringing your awareness back to the present moment. Gently open your eyes, carrying the balanced and authentic energy of the throat chakra with you into your interactions and communications as you go about your day.

• Note down any thoughts, feelings, observations, or ideas that came to you.

THROAT DAY 5: JOURNAL PROMPT

Engage in expressive writing exercises to tap into your voice and self-expression. Set aside time to journal, write poetry, or engage in stream-of-consciousness writing. Allow your thoughts and feelings to flow onto the paper without judgement. Explore your desires, dreams, and challenges through written expression. Leave the editor at the door! Play with what happens when you let your words fill the page.

THIRD EYE

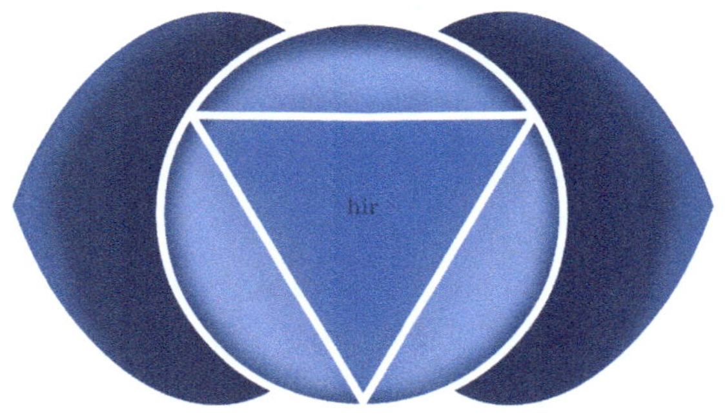

I see

THIRD EYE DAY 1: PHYSICAL ACTIVITY

The third eye chakra, located between the eyebrows, is associated with intuition, insight, and inner wisdom. When this energy centre is balanced, we feel connected to our higher selves and able to access deep truths and guidance from within. Engaging in physical activities that promote mental clarity, spiritual awareness, and inner reflection can help cultivate balance in the third eye chakra.

One powerful way to nurture the third eye chakra is to take yourself outside at night to gaze at the night sky. Stargazing is a profoundly awe-inspiring activity that can help to open and balance the third eye chakra, our centre of intuition, insight, and inner wisdom. With regular practice, stargazing can become a powerful tool for cultivating inner vision, expanding your consciousness, and aligning yourself with the infinite wisdom of the universe. And isn't it so lovely to have a good, healing reason for gazing up at the beautiful heavens?

Another physical activity that can help balance the third eye chakra is engaging in creative pursuits that require imagination and visualisation, such as painting, drawing, or sculpting. The process of bringing an inner vision to life through art can be a powerful way to access and express the wisdom of the third eye. As you create, focus on the images and ideas that arise from within, allowing them to flow through you onto the canvas or clay. Trust in the unique vision and perspective that you bring to your art, knowing that it is a reflection of your deepest truths and insights. It's not about perfection in artistry. It's about what is beautiful and moving to you.

Engaging in activities that challenge your mind and expand your perspective, such as solving puzzles, reading thought-provoking books, or attending lectures and workshops, can also be beneficial for the third eye chakra. By exposing yourself to new ideas and ways of thinking, you stimulate your mental faculties and open yourself up to new possibilities and insights. As you engage in these activities, approach them with a beginner's mind, letting go of preconceived notions and remaining open to the wisdom and knowledge that may arise.

As you explore these physical activities, remember to approach them with a spirit of curiosity, openness, and trust in your own inner guidance. Notice any doubts or fears that arise and gently acknowledge them, while also choosing to focus on the insights and wisdom that emerge from within. Celebrate the unique gifts and perspectives that you bring to the world, knowing that your intuition and inner vision are powerful tools for growth, healing, and transformation. Trust that by nurturing your third eye chakra through these practices, you are cultivating a deep sense of self-awareness, spiritual connection, and inner wisdom that will guide and support you on your journey.

Choose One of the Following Activities

Stargazing

Spend time observing the night sky, allowing a sense of wonder and connection to the universe to expand your perspective and intuition. On a clear night, find a quiet, dark location away from city lights, and allow yourself to settle into a comfortable position, either sitting or lying down. As you gaze up at the vast expanse of the night sky, let your eyes adjust to the darkness and begin to observe the countless stars, planets, and constellations above you. Take deep, slow breaths, and allow your mind to quiet, releasing any thoughts or worries that may arise. As you immerse yourself in the timeless beauty of the cosmos, notice any sensations of wonder, peace, or unity that arise within you. Allow yourself to contemplate the mysteries of the universe, the vastness of creation, and your own place within it. As you open yourself to the wisdom of the stars, trust that your third eye chakra is being activated and awakened, granting you access to deeper levels of intuition, clarity, and spiritual connection.

Intuitive Collage

Gather a variety of magazines, images, and art supplies, and find a quiet space to create. Take a few moments to centre yourself and connect with your intuition, setting an intention for the wisdom and insights you wish to receive. Then, begin flipping through the magazines, allowing yourself to be drawn to images and words that resonate with you on a deep level. Cut out the images and arrange them on a piece of paper or canvas, trusting your intuition to guide the placement and composition. Alternatively, use a digital forum, like Pinterest or Canva, to collate all the pictures, quotes, and visions you love. When your collage feels complete, take a step back and observe it with fresh eyes, noticing any themes, messages, or insights that emerge.

Attend a Mind-Expanding Workshop

Research local workshops, lectures, or classes on topics that interest you and expand your perspective, such as philosophy, spirituality, science, or psychology. Choose an event that resonates with you and attend with an open mind and a willingness to learn. As you listen to the presenter and engage in discussions with other attendees, notice any new ideas or insights that arise, and allow yourself to be challenged and inspired by different viewpoints. After the event, take some time to reflect on your experience, journaling about any key takeaways or questions that emerged.

THIRD EYE DAY 1: JOURNAL PROMPT

How do I connect with my intuition and inner wisdom? Reflect on moments when you've trusted your intuition and made decisions based on inner guidance. How did it transpire, and how do you feel this turned out? How can you cultivate a deeper connection with your intuition and honour the wisdom of your Third Eye Chakra?

Third Eye Day 2: Food, Drink, Herbs, & Spices

Today we're going to support our third eye chakra, the Ajna, nutritionally. The third eye is our centre of intuition, wisdom, and inner vision. Between the eyebrows, this energy centre is associated with our ability to see beyond the physical realm, to access our inner guidance and higher knowledge, and to perceive the world with clarity and insight. When the third eye chakra is balanced, we feel a deep sense of connection to our intuition and inner wisdom. We trust our instincts, see beyond appearances and illusions, and navigate life's challenges with a sense of purpose and direction. We are open to new ideas and perspectives, and we are able to integrate our experiences into a larger understanding of ourselves and the world around us.

To support this sense of intuitive wisdom and clarity in the third eye chakra, it's important to focus on foods and drinks that are nourishing, cleansing, and energetically uplifting. These foods tend to be rich in antioxidants, omega-3 fatty acids, and other nutrients that support brain health and cognitive function, while also promoting a sense of mental clarity and spiritual awareness.

Some specific foods that can be particularly supportive of the third eye chakra include:

Blueberries: Blueberries are rich in antioxidants and other nutrients that support brain health and cognitive function. They have been shown to improve memory, focus, and overall mental clarity, making them a great choice for those seeking to enhance their intuitive abilities and inner vision. Try enjoying blueberries on their own as a snack, or adding them to smoothies, oatmeal, or yogurt.

Omega-3 Rich Foods: Omega-3 fatty acids are essential for brain health and cognitive function, and they have been shown to support mental clarity, emotional balance, and overall well-being. Good sources of omega-3s include fatty fish like salmon, sardines, and mackerel, as well as plant-based sources like chia seeds, flax seeds, and walnuts. Try incorporating these foods into your diet on a regular basis to support your third eye chakra.

Dark Leafy Greens: Dark leafy greens like spinach, kale, and collard greens are packed with vitamins, minerals, and antioxidants that support brain health and overall vitality. They are also rich in chlorophyll, a natural detoxifier that can help to cleanse the body and promote mental clarity. Try incorporating dark leafy greens into your diet as a salad, a sautéed side dish, or a smoothie ingredient.

Purple Foods: In chakra theory, the colour purple is associated with the third eye chakra, and eating foods that are naturally purple in colour can help to stimulate and balance this energy centre. Good options include purple cabbage, purple carrots, and acai berries. These foods are also rich in antioxidants and other nutrients that support brain health and spiritual awareness.

Herbal Teas: Certain herbal teas are particularly supportive of the third eye chakra, thanks to their ability to promote mental clarity, relaxation, and spiritual awareness. Good options include chamomile, lavender, and passionflower tea, as well as teas made with ginkgo biloba, a herb that has been shown to improve memory and cognitive function. Try enjoying a cup of herbal tea in the evening as a soothing and uplifting ritual.

In addition to these specific foods and drinks, it's important to focus on eating a balanced and nourishing diet that supports your overall health and well-being. Aim to incorporate a variety of fresh, whole foods into your meals, and limit your intake of processed, sugary, and artificial foods, which can be draining and depleting to the third eye chakra. When it comes to drinks, water is once again a key component of a third eye chakra-balancing diet. Aim to drink plenty of pure, clean water throughout the day, and consider adding a slice of lemon or a sprig of mint for an extra boost of cleansing and energising power.

Other beverages that can be supportive for the third eye chakra include green tea and matcha, which are rich in antioxidants and other nutrients that support brain health and mental clarity. You may also want to experiment with adaptogenic herbs like ashwagandha, lion's mane, and gotu kola, which can help to promote mental clarity, reduce stress and anxiety, and support overall cognitive function.

As with the other chakras, it's important to approach your third eye chakra-balancing diet with mindfulness and self-awareness. Pay attention to how different foods and drinks make you feel, both physically

and energetically, and trust your own inner guidance when it comes
to making choices that support your unique needs and goals.

> ## Purple Foods, Drinks, Herbs, & Spices

Purple grapes and grape juice, purple kale, blueberries, purple cabbage, aubergine, and purple carrots. Coconut oil, water, beautiful dark
green-blue spirulina. Use the herbs rosemary and lavender, passionflower and sage. Please also include cacao and dark chocolate!

A Third Eye Chakra Infusion

- 2 sprigs of fresh lavender with flowers
- 1 teaspoon dried lavender
- 2 sprigs of fresh rosemary
- 400ml hot boiled water

Let all infuse for 5 minutes. You can drink this hot, or let it
cool and have it at room temperature, chilled, or over ice, if you
prefer. Strain, and pour into your favourite mug or glass, and
then make a ritual of drinking it.

An alternative third eye chakra drink

Treat yourself to some ceremonial grade cacao powder and/or
nibs. Gently heat your choice of milk in a pan, and add the
cacao. When it's melted, add raw honey or your favourite natural
sweetener. Whisk gently. Fill the pan with love, being mindful of
the intention you are setting with this ceremony.

Sip slowly and mindfully, absorbing the prayers you added.

THIRD EYE DAY 2: JOURNAL PROMPT

What dreams or visions have I experienced that hold significance? Reflect on any dreams or visions you've had that felt profound or held symbolic meaning. Explore the messages or insights they may have contained and how they relate to your life.

THIrD EYE DAY 3: YOGA

We are back to the yoga part of this chakra balancing work. As you know, the third eye chakra, also known as Ajna, is the sixth energy centre, located between the eyebrows. It is associated with our ability to see clearly, both in the physical world and in the realm of intuition and inner wisdom. When this chakra is balanced and open, we feel a strong sense of insight, clarity, and connection to our higher purpose and spiritual path. Yoga can help us to release physical and mental tension, cultivate a sense of focus and concentration, and connect with our inner source of wisdom and guidance.

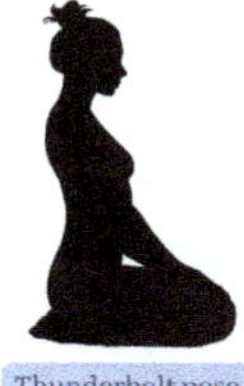
Thunderbolt pose
(Vajrasana)

One of the most effective poses for the third eye chakra is Thunderbolt Pose (Vajrasana), and it's such a simple one! This simple seated posture helps to calm the mind and promotes a sense of grounding and stability in the body. As you sit back on your heels with your spine straight and your hands resting on your thighs, you allow stillness, and a sense of focus in the third eye chakra. This opens you up to feeling inner peace and clarity.

Head-to-Knee Pose (Janu Sirsasana) is a gentle forward bend that helps to release tension in the spine and hips, while also promoting a sense of introspection and self-reflection. As you fold forward over one leg, keeping the other leg extended, you allow a sense of surrender and re-

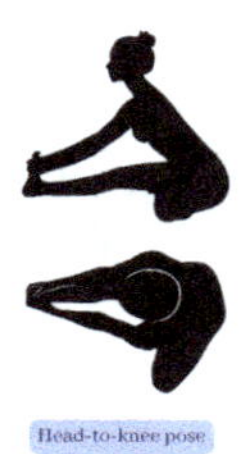

Head-to-knee pose
(Janu Sirsasana)

ceptivity in the third eye centre, letting a feeling of inner wisdom and intuition develop.

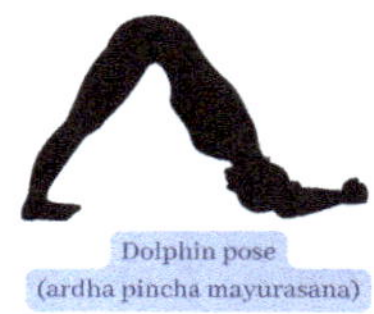

Dolphin pose
(ardha pincha mayurasana)

Dolphin Pose (Ardha Pincha Mayurasana) is a strengthening and stretching posture that can help to build upper body strength and flexibility, while also promoting a sense of focus and concentration in the mind. As you lift your hips and lengthen your spine, supporting yourself with your forearms and elbows, weyoucreate a sense of balance and alignment in your third eye chakra, developing clarity and insight.

Extended Child's Pose (Utthita Balasana) is a gentle resting posture that can help to release tension in the back and hips, while also encouraging introspection and self-reflection. This is a lovely pose to do at the end of the day, especially if your day has involved a lot of sitting. As you extend your arms forward and allow your forehead to rest on the ground (or a cushion, if that is more comfortable), you create a sense of surrender and receptivity in the third eye chakra, allowing a feeling of inner wisdom and guidance.

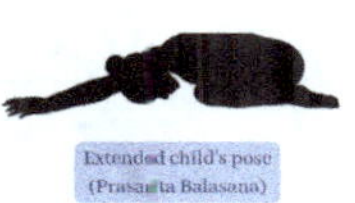
Extended child's pose
(Prasarita Balasana)

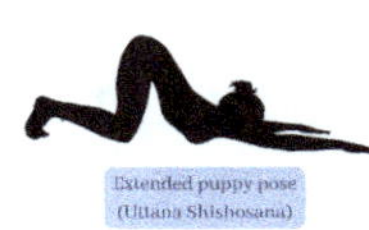
Extended puppy pose
(Uttana Shishosana)

Extended Puppy Pose (Uttana Shishosana) is a gentle backbend that helps to open the chest and shoulders, allowing a sense of focus and concentration in the mind. As you keep your hips lifted and your forehead resting on the ground, you enable a sense of balance and alignment in the third eye centre, promoting a feeling of clarity and insight.

Half Forward Fold (Ardha Uttanasana) is a gentle forward bend that helps to stretch the spine and hamstrings, while also enabling a sense of introspection and self-reflection. As you fold forward from the hips, keeping your spine long and your shoulders relaxed, you create a sense of surrender and receptivity in the third eye chakra, encouraging a feeling of inner wisdom and intuition.

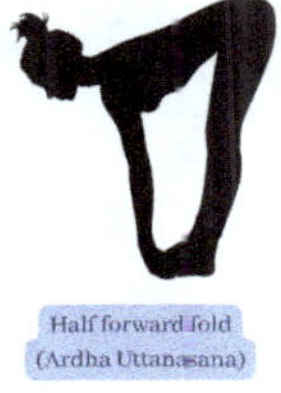
Half forward fold
(Ardha Uttanasana)

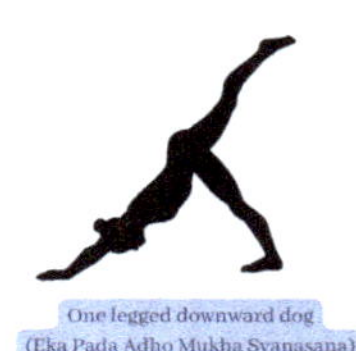

One legged downward dog
(Eka Pada Adho Mukha Svanasana)

Finally, One-Legged Downward Dog (Eka Pada Adho Mukha Svanasana) is a challenging balance posture that can help to build strength and flexibility in the legs and spine, while also encouraging a sense of focus and concentration in the mind. As you lift one leg towards the sky and keep the other leg strong and grounded, you create a sense of balance and alignment in the third eye centre, allowing a feeling of clarity and insight.

Incorporating these poses into a regular yoga practice can help to balance and activate the third eye chakra, promoting a sense of intuition, clarity, and connection to our inner wisdom and higher purpose. However, it is important to approach these poses with mindfulness and self-compassion, honouring your body's unique needs and limitations. In addition to the physical benefits, yoga for the third eye chakra also offers profound mental and spiritual benefits. By connecting with our inner source of wisdom and intuition, we can cultivate a greater sense of self-awareness, self-trust, and self-guidance. We can learn to see clearly through the distractions and illusions of the mind, and to align ourselves with our true path and purpose.

THIRD EYE DAY 3: JOURNAL PROMPT

How can I cultivate a sense of clarity and mental focus? As you write, explore other practices that help you cultivate mental clarity and focus, such as meditation or mindfulness. Reflect on strategies that can support your ability to see situations with clarity and discernment. How do you reduce the clutter and noise of daily life?

THIRD EYE DAY 4: EFT

EFT tapping, short for Emotional Freedom Techniques, is a therapeutic technique that combines gentle tapping on specific acupressure points on the body with focused attention on emotional issues. It aims to release emotional blockages and restore balance in the body's energy system. By tapping on these points while acknowledging and addressing emotional concerns, EFT tapping can help alleviate stress, anxiety, and other negative emotions, promoting a sense of emotional well-being.

You begin with a set-up statement, which you repeat three times whilst tapping on the karate chop point. You then repeat an affirmation whilst tapping gently on each tapping point in turn. Don't worry about remembering everything, this page is repeated for each chakra!

Tapping points

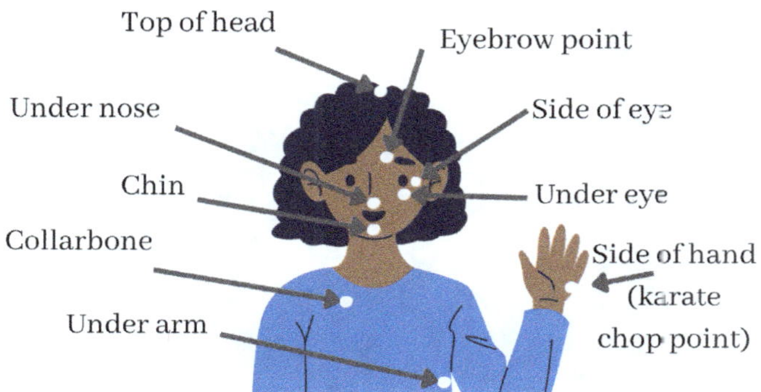

Set up phrase - tap side of hand (karate chop point):

"Even though I don't trust my intuition, I love and accept myself.

Even though I've got a lot to learn, I love myself exactly as I am now.

Even though I am not always connected to my higher guidance, I love, honour and accept myself completely."

Eyebrow point: "I trust my intuition and follow its guidance with clarity and confidence."

Side of eye: "I am connected to my inner wisdom and make decisions from a place of deep knowing."

Under eye: "I see beyond the physical realm and perceive the hidden truths of the universe."

Under nose: "I embrace my inner vision and manifest my dreams into reality."

Chin: "I cultivate a clear and focused mind, free from distractions and limiting beliefs."

Collarbone: "I am open to receiving divine insights and messages from the higher realms."

Under arm: "I trust in the process of life and surrender to the flow of the universe."

Top of head: "I am in tune with the greater picture of my life, finding meaning and purpose in every experience."

Repeat seven times.

THIRD EYE DAY 4: JOURNAL PROMPT

How can I balance my analytical thinking with intuitive knowing? Reflect on the balance between analytical thinking and intuitive knowing in your life. Do you lean more one way or the other? Are there situations where one is more helpful? Explore ways to integrate both approaches, allowing for a harmonious blend of logic and intuition.

THIRD EYE DAY 5: CRYSTALS & MEDITATION

I f you have one of these crystals, hold it while you follow this meditation. If you don't have one, don't worry. You can hold a picture of one, or simply visualise on in your hands as you meditate. If you'd like me to lead you in this meditation, you can go to my store and download it for free, or find me under Jennifer Jones on the meditation app Insight Timer.

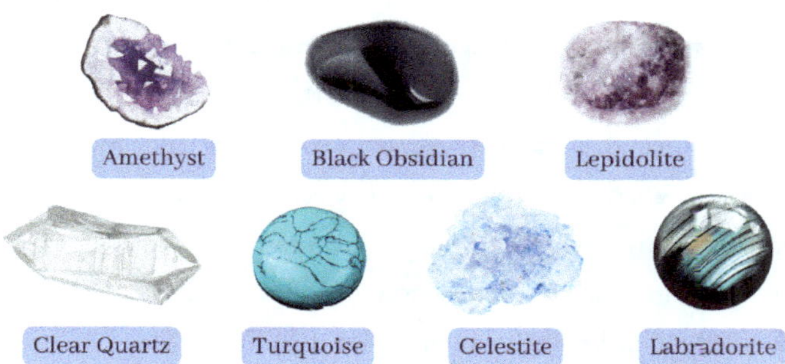

• Find a quiet and comfortable space where you can sit or lie down without distractions. Close your eyes and take a few deep breaths, allowing your body and mind to relax.

• Visualise a deep indigo light in the centre of your forehead, where the third eye chakra is located. See this light growing brighter with each breath, expanding to fill your entire forehead with soothing and illuminating energy.

• Imagine the indigo light swirling and spinning in a clockwise direction, clearing any blockages or stagnant energy within the third eye chakra. Feel a sense of clarity and heightened awareness emanating from this energy centre.

• As this indigo light swirls through you, visualise it filling and connecting every cell of your body. See yourself connected to each part of yourself, able to communicate and receive wisdom from your own inner guidance, however that shows up for you. • Expand your awareness beyond the physical realm. Imagine yourself connecting with the vastness of the universe, opening your mind to receive divine knowledge and wisdom. Embrace the infinite possibilities and pro-found insights that reside within you.

• Observe any emotions or feelings that rise up as you. Note them without judgment, but accept yourself exactly as you are. Let any questions you have form in your mind, and release any expectation of an answer. Trust that whatever wisdom you receive in this space is exactly what is intended for you right at this moment.

• Remain in this healing energy of the third eye chakra for as long as you want. When you're ready take a few deep breaths, gradually bringing your awareness back to the present moment. Gently open your eyes, and carry the heightened awareness and spiritual connection of the third eye chakra with you into your daily life.

• Note down any thoughts, feelings, observations, or ideas that came to you.

THIRD EYE DAY 5: JOURNAL PROMPT

Reflect on moments when you've experienced heightened intuition or psychic insights. How did it feel? How can you further develop and trust these abilities? Try automatic writing, or pulling a tarot or oracle card and writing about what comes up for you.

CROWN

I know

crown Day 1: PHYSICaL ACTIVITY

The crown chakra, located at the top of the head, is associated with spiritual connection, enlightenment, and unity consciousness. When this energy centre is balanced, we feel a deep sense of oneness with the universe and a profound understanding of our true nature as spiritual beings. Engaging in physical activities that promote inner stillness, divine connection, and a sense of transcendence can help cultivate balance in the crown chakra.

One powerful way to nurture the crown chakra is through the practice of mindfulness and present-moment awareness. By bringing our attention fully into the here and now, we create space for the wisdom and insight of the divine to flow through us. Whether you choose to practice mindfulness through seated meditation, walking in nature, or simply bringing a sense of presence to your daily activities, the act of being fully awake and aware in each moment can be incredibly transformative. As you practice mindfulness, imagine a pure, white light streaming down from the heavens, entering your crown chakra, and filling your entire being with a sense of peace, clarity, and connection.

Chanting is a powerful tool for activating and balancing the crown chakra. By engaging in the repetition of sacred sounds or mantras, we create a vibrational frequency that resonates with the crown chakra, helping to open and align this energy centre. As we chant, we quiet the mind, release attachments to the ego, and cultivate a deep sense of oneness with the universe. Regular chanting can lead to profound experiences of inner stillness, expanded awareness, and spiritual awakening, as we tap into the infinite wisdom and love that resides within us all. By incorporating chanting into our spiritual practice, we support the healthy functioning of the crown chakra, allowing us to live with greater purpose, meaning, and connection to the divine.

Engaging in activities that promote a sense of awe, wonder, and reverence for the mystery of life can also be beneficial for the crown chakra. Spending time in nature, gazing at the stars, or contemplating the vastness of the universe can help us connect with something greater than ourselves and tap into the wisdom of the divine. As you engage in these activities, allow yourself to be filled with a sense of humility, gratitude, and reverence for the beauty and complexity of creation. Trust that by opening yourself to the mystery and grandeur of life, you are aligning yourself with the highest wisdom and guidance available.

As you explore these physical activities, remember to approach them with a sense of surrender, trust, and openness to the divine. Let go of any expectations or attachments to specific outcomes, and allow yourself to be guided by the wisdom and insight that arises from within. Celebrate the moments of connection, clarity, and transcendence that emerge, knowing that they are reflections of your true nature as a spiritual being. Trust that by nurturing your crown chakra through these practices, you are cultivating a deep sense of unity, purpose, and connection with the divine that will guide and support you on your journey.

Choose One of the Following Activities

Mindful Nature Immersion

Find a peaceful natural setting, such as a park, beach, or forest, and allow yourself to fully immerse in the beauty and tranquility of your surroundings. As you walk or sit in nature, bring your attention to the present moment, noticing the sights, sounds, smells, and sensations that arise. Let go of any thoughts or worries about the past or future, and simply allow yourself to be fully present with the natural world around you. As you deepen into a state of mindful awareness, notice any sensations of peace, unity, or divine connection that arise.

Chanting

Find a comfortable seated position in a quiet, peaceful space. Close your eyes, and take a few deep, centring breaths, allowing your body to relax and your mind to become still. Choose a mantra or sacred phrase that resonates with you, such as "Om," "So Hum," or "Sat Nam," and begin to repeat it out loud, allowing the sound to vibrate through your entire being. As you chant, bring your awareness to the top of your head, visualizing a pure, white light entering your crown chakra and filling your entire being with a sense of peace, clarity, and divine connection. Let go of any thoughts or distractions that arise, and simply allow yourself to be fully immersed in the sound and vibration of the chant. As you continue to chant, notice any sensations of expansion, lightness, or transcendence that arise within you. Trust that with each repetition, you are strengthening your connection to the divine, opening yourself to higher levels of consciousness, and aligning yourself with the infinite wisdom and love of the universe. With regular practice, chanting can become a transformative tool for awakening your crown chakra, deepening your spiritual understanding, and cultivating a profound sense of unity and oneness with all that is.

Attend a Spiritual Retreat or Workshop

Research local or online spiritual retreats, workshops, or events that focus on themes of unity, enlightenment, or divine connection. Choose an event that resonates with you and attend with an open heart and mind, setting an intention to deepen your spiritual understanding and awareness. As you participate in the various activities and teachings offered, allow yourself to fully embrace the experience, letting go of any resistance or preconceived notions. Notice any moments of insight, clarity, or transcendence that arise, and trust in the wisdom and guidance that is being revealed to you.

Crown Day 1: Journal Prompt

How do I connect with the divine or higher power in my life? Reflect on your connection with the divine or higher power. Explore your spiritual beliefs, practices, and experiences that foster a sense of connection and transcendence.

crown Day 2: Foods, Drinks, Herbs, & Spices

Let's consider how we can nutritionally support the final chakra in our journey of exploration: the crown chakra, or Sahasrara, the centre of spiritual connection, unity consciousness, and divine wisdom. Located at the top of the head, this ethereal energy centre is associated with our ability to transcend the limitations of the ego and connect with the infinite source of all creation. When the crown chakra is balanced, we feel a profound sense of oneness and interconnectedness with all beings. We are able to let go of our attachments to the material world and our limited sense of self, and to rest in the pure awareness of our true nature. We experience a deep sense of peace, joy, and fulfilment that comes from aligning with our highest purpose and living in harmony with the universe.

To support this sense of spiritual connection and unity in the crown chakra, it's important to focus on foods and drinks that are pure, light, and energetically uplifting. These foods tend to be rich in prana, or life force energy, and have a subtle yet powerful effect on our consciousness and spiritual awareness.

Some specific foods that can be particularly supportive for the crown chakra include:

Fresh Fruits & Vegetables: Fresh, organic fruits and vegetables are rich in prana and have a naturally purifying and uplifting effect on the body and mind. They are also rich in vitamins, minerals, and antioxidants that support overall health and vitality. Try incorporating a variety of colourful fruits and vegetables into your diet, with an emphasis on leafy greens, berries, and other nutrient-dense foods.

Pure Water: Pure, clean water is essential for the health and function of all the chakras, but it is especially important for the crown chakra. Water has a naturally purifying and cleansing effect on the body and mind, and can help to clear away any blocked or stagnant energy in the crown chakra. What a blessing that we live in a time when clean water is available to us! Aim to drink plenty of pure, filtered water throughout the day, and consider adding a few drops of lemon or lime juice for an extra boost of cleansing power.

Herbal Teas: Certain herbal teas can be particularly supportive of the crown chakra, thanks to their ability to promote mental clarity, spiritual awareness, and inner peace. Good options include chamomile, lavender, and rose tea, as well as teas made with holy basil (tulsi), gotu kola, and ginkgo biloba. Try enjoying a cup of herbal tea in the morning or evening as a soothing and uplifting ritual.

Raw Cacao: Raw cacao is a powerful superfood that is rich in antioxidants, magnesium, and other nutrients that support brain health and spiritual awareness. It is also a natural source of theobromine, a compound that has a gentle stimulating effect on the mind and can help to promote mental clarity and focus. Try incorporating raw cacao into your diet in the form of cacao nibs, cacao powder, or raw chocolate.

Fasting & Cleansing: Fasting and cleansing can be powerful tools for supporting the health and balance of the crown chakra, as they help to purify the body and mind and create space for spiritual growth and transformation. You could try incorporating short periods of fasting or cleansing into your routine, such as a one-day juice fast or a three-day raw food cleanse. It's also just as beneficial to simply consciously abstain from eating for a period of time – maybe choose to skip breakfast and extend your natural overnight fast, or make the decision to limit your evening snacking. Be sure to listen to your body and consult with a healthcare professional before undertaking any significant dietary changes.

In addition to these specific foods and practices, it's important to focus on cultivating a sense of mindfulness and presence in your eating and drinking habits. Take the time to sit down and enjoy your meals in a relaxed and peaceful setting, free from distractions and stress. Practice gratitude and appreciation for the food and drink you consume, and take a moment to offer a silent blessing or intention before each meal. It's also important to be mindful of any patterns of emotional eating or using food as a means of distraction or avoidance. The crown chakra is associated with our ability to let go of attachments and rest in the pure awareness of the present moment, and this includes letting go of any unhealthy attachments to food or other external substances.

Remember that true spiritual connection and unity come from within, and that no external substance or experience can replace the power of your own inner wisdom and divine nature. By nourishing your body with pure, uplifting foods and drinks, and by cultivating a deep sense of presence and awareness in your daily life, you can support a healthy and balanced crown chakra, and experience the profound sense of peace, joy, and oneness that is your birthright.

Foods, Drinks, Herbs, & Spices

To nurture and balance this chakra, many people choose to fast, or to eat very lightly. It is a good time to recognise that food is a gift, and to give thanks for it before each meal We can also be mindful of the quality of our food, and the impact it has on our bodies and on the world around us. You could choose to take nourishing broths or herby infusions to help detoxify the body and lighten the load for the intestines, as you spend time in prayer or meditation. The following ingredients could help:

Sage, chamomile, saffron, frankincense, and juniper.

A Crown Chakra Infusion

- •1 slice of organic lemon with peel
- • 1 teaspoon dried sage
- • 400ml hot boiled water

Let all infuse for 5 minutes. You can drink this hot, or let it cool and have it at room temperature, chilled, or over ice, if you prefer. Strain, and pour into your favourite mug or glass, and then make a ritual of drinking it.

An alternative crown chakra dish

Prepare a light vegetable broth, with turmeric, garlic and ginger to cleanse and detoxify. Prepare with intention, noticing the scents, colours and shapes of each ingredient, and acknowledging how they came from their place of origin to your home. Set your table consciously, and eat with gratitude.

Crown Day 2: Journal Prompt

What brings me a sense of awe and wonder? Reflect on experiences or moments that have evoked a deep sense of awe and wonder within you. What aspects of life or the universe ignite your curiosity and expand your consciousness?

Crown Day 3: Yoga

We've reached our final yoga day in this series of chakra balancing practices. The crown chakra, also known as Sahasrara, is, of course, the seventh and highest energy centre, located at the top of the head. It is associated with our ability to connect with the divine, experience unity consciousness, and realise our true nature as spiritual beings. When this chakra is balanced and open, we feel a deep sense of peace, joy, and oneness with all of creation. As with all the chakras, yoga offers a powerful set of tools for balancing and activating the crown chakra. By incorporating specific poses into our practice, we can help to release physical and mental tensions, cultivate a sense of inner stillness and presence, and connect with our highest truth and purpose.

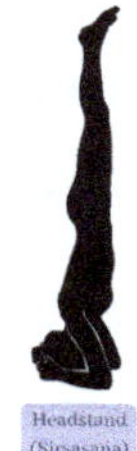

Headstand
(Sirsasana)

One of the most effective poses for the crown chakra is Headstand (Sirsasana). Please only attempt this if you are physically confident of standing on your head! This challenging inversion helps to stimulate the crown chakra by bringing fresh blood and oxygen to the brain, while also encouraging a sense of focus, concentration, and inner stillness. As you balance on the crown of your head with your hands supporting your body, you create a sense of alignment and connection with the divine, promoting a feeling of spiritual awakening and enlightenment.

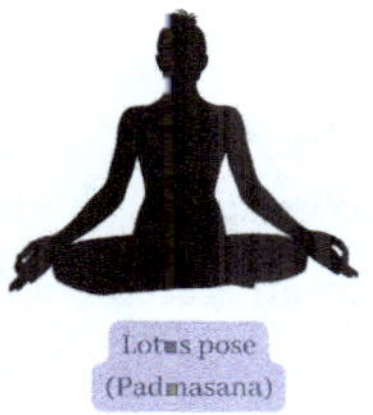

Lotus pose
(Padmasana)

Lotus Pose (Padmasana) is a classic meditation posture that helps to calm the mind, and promotes a sense of inner peace and tranquility. As you sit with your legs crossed and your spine straight, you create a sense of stability and groundedness in the body, while also opening the hips and allowing the energy to flow freely through all the chakras up to the crown chakra, allowing a feeling of spiritual connection and unity.

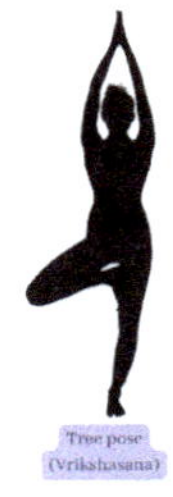
Tree pose
(Vrikshasana)

Tree Pose (Vrksasana) is a balancing posture that helps to cultivate a sense of inner strength, stability, and focus. As you stand on one leg with your other foot resting on your inner thigh or calf, you create a sense of rootedness and connection with the earth, while also lifting the energy up through the body to the crown chakra, promoting a feeling of spiritual growth and expansion.

Camel Pose (Ustrasana) is a deep backbend that helps to open the chest and shoulders, while also stimulating the thyroid and pituitary glands, which are closely associated with the crown chakra. As you kneel on the floor and reach back to grasp your heels, you create a sense of surrender and receptivity in your heart centre, while also allowing the energy to flow freely up to the crown chakra, embracing a feeling of spiritual awakening and liberation.

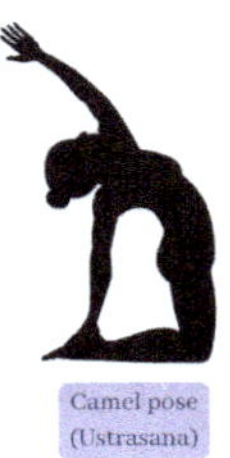
Camel pose
(Ustrasana)

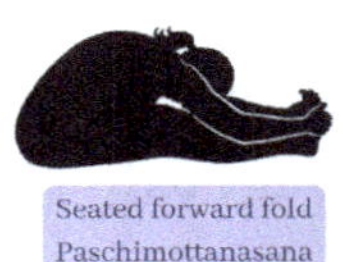
Seated forward fold
Paschimottanasana

Seated Forward Fold (Paschimottanasana) is a gentle forward bend that helps to calm the mind and promote a sense of introspection and self-reflection. You don't need to force it, but just let yourself relax forward as far as you can comfortably go. As you fold forward over your legs with your spine straight and your head relaxed, you create a sense of surrender and letting go, while also allowing the energy to flow freely up to the crown chakra, promoting a feeling of spiritual connection and inner peace.

Cow Face Pose (Gomukhasana) is a deep hip opener that can help to release physical and emotional tensions, while also promoting a sense of inner awareness and self-discovery. This pose can be quite intense, so be gentle with yourself and pause or stop if you need to. As you sit with one

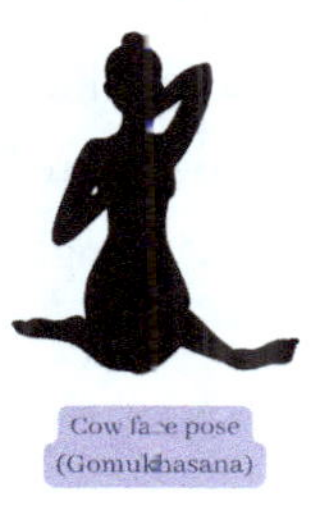

Cow face pose (Gomukhasana)

knee stacked on top of the other, and your arms clasped behind your back, you create a sense of balance and alignment in your body, while also allowing the energy to flow freely up to the crown chakra. Enjoy this feeling of spiritual awakening and self-realisation.

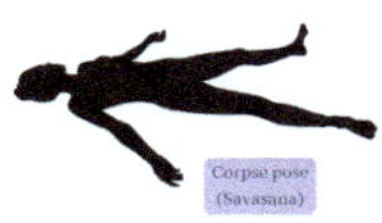

Corpse pose (Savasana)

Finally, Corpse Pose (Savasana) is a deeply restful and rejuvenating posture that integrates all the benefits of the practice and leaves you with a sense of inner peace and connection with the divine. Lie on your back with your arms and legs relaxed and your eyes closed. Breathe naturally, surrender, let go. Allow the energy to flow freely through your body, bathing every chakra. Let yourself absorb this feeling of spiritual unity and oneness.

Incorporating these poses into a regular yoga practice can help to balance and activate the crown chakra, and all chakras, encouraging a sense of spiritual connection, inner peace, and unity consciousness. However, please approach these poses with mindfulness and self-compassion, honouring your unique body's needs and limitations. In addition to the physical benefits, yoga for the crown chakra also offers profound spiritual and existential benefits. By connecting with our highest truth and purpose, we can cultivate a greater sense of meaning, fulfilment, and inner peace in our lives. We learn to let go of the ego's limited perspective and embrace the vast, infinite nature of our true being.

Crown Day 3: Journal Prompt

How can I cultivate a sense of surrender and trust in the unfolding of life? Explore the concept of surrender and trust in relation to the divine plan or the greater flow of life. Reflect on ways you can let go of control and cultivate a deep trust in the unfolding of your journey.

Crown Day 4: EFT

EFT tapping, short for Emotional Freedom Techniques, is a therapeutic technique that combines gentle tapping on specific acupressure points on the body with focused attention on emotional issues. It aims to release emotional blockages and restore balance in the body's energy system. By tapping on these points while acknowledging and addressing emotional concerns, EFT tapping can help alleviate stress, anxiety, and other negative emotions, promoting a sense of emotional well-being.

You begin with a set-up statement, which you repeat three times whilst tapping on the karate chop point. You then repeat an affirmation whilst tapping gently on each tapping point in turn. Don't worry about remembering everything, this page is repeated for each chakra!

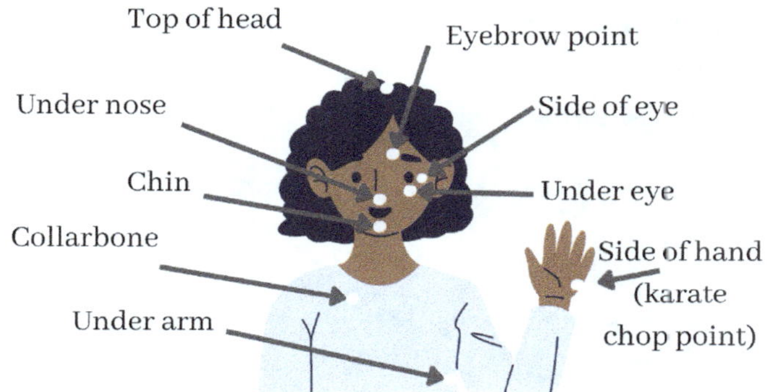

Set up phrase - tap side of hand (karate chop point):

"Even though I'm feeling disconnected from source, I love and accept myself.

Even though I've got a lot to learn, I love myself exactly as I am now.

Even though I don't trust that I know my purpose in life, I love, honour and accept myself completely."

Eyebrow point: "I am connected to the divine energy that flows through all things."

Side of eye: "I embrace my spiritual essence and trust in the higher wisdom of the universe."

Under eye: "I am open to receiving divine guidance and inspiration."

Under nose: "I am a vessel for divine love, light, and wisdom to flow through me."

Chin: "I surrender to the divine intelligence and trust in the unfolding of my life's journey."

Collarbone: "I am aligned with the infinite possibilities of the universe."

Under arm: "I am one with the universal consciousness, experiencing unity and oneness with all."

Top of head: "I am a divine being, here to shine my unique light and make a positive impact in the world."

Repeat seven times.

Crown Day 4: Journal Prompt

What practices or rituals nourish my soul and expand my consciousness? Reflect on practices or rituals that nurture your soul and expand your consciousness. Explore meditation, prayer, nature walks, or any other practices that bring you closer to the divine. How do these make you feel connected?

Crown Day : Crystals & Meditation

If you have one of these crystals, hold it while you follow this meditation. If you don't have one, don't worry. You can hold a picture of one, or simply visualise on in your hands as you meditate. If you'd like me to lead you in this meditation, you can go to my store and download it for free, or find me under Jennifer Jones on the meditation app Insight Timer.

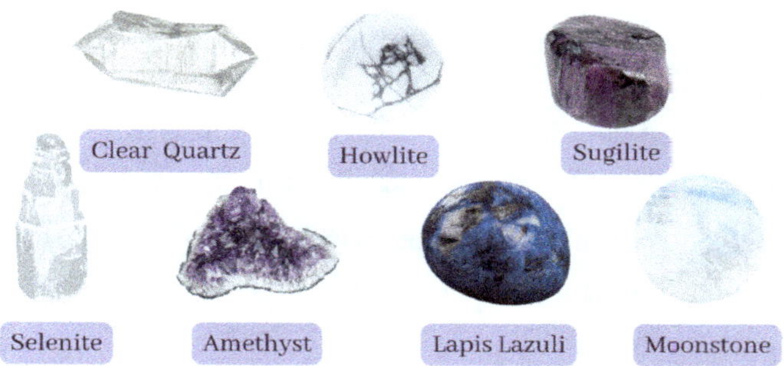

• Find a quiet and comfortable space where you can sit or lie down without distractions. Close your eyes and take a few deep breaths, allowing your body and mind to relax.

• Visualise a luminous violet light at the top of your head, where the crown chakra is located. Feel the warmth of this light opening your crown chakra, enveloping your skull, head and aura with divine and transcendent energy.

• The violet light swirls gently and spins in a clockwise direction, clearing any blockages or stagnant energy within the crown chakra. Feel a sense of openness and connection to the divine flowing from this energy centre.

• Allow this warmth to spread down through each chakra and let the energy vibrate all the way through the root and into the earth, securing you to earth energy.

• Bring your awareness to the area above your head and beyond the physical realm. Imagine a golden beam of light descending from above, symbolising divine energy and guidance. Feel this golden light entering through the top of your head, illuminating your entire being and connecting you to the vastness of the universe. You are aligned with divine wisdom and able to access universal knowledge, feeling all-that-is flowing through you.

• Remain in this connected energy for as long as you want. When you're ready to return, take a few deep breaths, gradually bringing your awareness back to the present moment. Move your fingers and toes, and thank the universe for any wisdom you may have received. Gently open your eyes, carrying the expanded consciousness and spiritual connection of the crown chakra with you into your daily life.

• Note down any thoughts, feelings, observations, or ideas that came to you.

crown Day 5: Journal Prompt

How can I cultivate a sense of unity and interconnectedness with all beings? Reflect on the concept of unity and interconnectedness. Explore ways to embrace a sense of oneness with all beings and the world around you. How can you cultivate compassion, empathy, and a sense of shared humanity?

Conclusion

Congratulations on completing your 35-day journey of chakra balancing!! You made it! If you've come this far, you have just completed 35 days of self work. You've invested time in your physical, emotional, mental, spiritual, and energetic health. You've learned some new tools, or practiced long-forgotten ones. You've developed practical tools that you can add to your toolbox for the future. You've balanced your energies, listened to your body, paid attention in places you might have pushed through before. Through your dedication and commitment to these daily practices, you have taken a significant step towards greater self-awareness, emotional well-being, and spiritual growth. I hope you feel accomplished, proud, happy, and balanced!

As you reflect on your experiences over the past weeks, take a moment to celebrate the progress you've made and the insights you've gained. Remember that the path of chakra balancing is an ongoing journey, and the practices you've learned will continue to support and guide you in your daily life. Keep in mind that each of us is unique, and our paths to balance and harmony may differ. Trust your intuition and continue to explore the practices that resonate most deeply with you. Some people repeat the whole 35 day process every year, while others listen to their energies and take time to attune the individual chakras that feel misaligned. Perhaps you'll do a week of yoga, with a day for each chakra, or maybe a week of focussed meditation. Hopefully, you've found a new activity that will enrich your life from here on in! Gardening, or dance classes, writing, public speaking, or kickboxing might be new passions that you want to continue exploring. However you move on, be patient and compassionate with yourself, knowing that growth and transformation happen in their own perfect time.

As you move forward, remember to bring a sense of joy, curiosity, and lightheartedness to your continued practice. Embrace the ebbs and flows of your journey, and trust that every experience, whether challenging or uplifting, is an opportunity for learning and growth. Most importantly, know that the true essence of chakra balancing lies not in achieving a state of perfection, but in cultivating a deeper sense of self-love, authenticity, and connection to the world around you. By nurturing your own inner light, you not only bring greater balance and harmony to your own life but also radiate that positive energy to all those you encounter.

So, as you close this chapter of your journey, do so with a grateful heart and a renewed commitment to your own growth and well-being. Celebrate the beautiful, vibrant being that you are, and trust in the unfolding of your unique path. Remember, the practices you've learned will always be available to you, like dear friends, ready to support and guide you whenever you need them.

Thank you for embarking on this transformative journey of chakra balancing with me. May the insights and experiences you've gained continue to illuminate your path, and may you always find joy, purpose, and connection in the unfolding of your own sacred journey.

With love and light,
Jenny

ABOUT THE AUTHOR

Jenny Douglas is a multi-genre author, astrologer, and energy healing practitioner. She lives in Northumberland, UK, with her husband, four children, and a bonkers dog, and when she's not writing magical fantasy stories for children, penning time travel books for adults, exploring all aspects of spirituality, healing modalities, and the stars, you'll probably find her endlessly picking stuff up off the floor and wondering how the piles on the stairs are mysteriously invisible to everybody else in the house...

Jenny loves to hear from her readers! To get in touch, please visit www.inkystars.com or email her directly at jen@inkystars.com

ALSO BY

Books by Jenny Douglas

Spiritual Non-Fiction:
Chakras: A 35 Day Chakra Balancing Journal
The Manifestor's Workbook: A Journal For Manifestors in the Human Design System
The Generator's Workbook: A Journal for Generators in the Human Design System
The Manifesting Generator's Workbook: A Journal For Manifesting Generators in the Human Design System
The Projector's Workbook: A Journal For Projectors in the Human Design System
The Reflector's Workbook: A Journal For Reflectors in the Human Design System

Books by Jen Jones

Middle Grade Fiction – ages 9-12:
The Merryshields Series

Merryshields: The Island In The Attic

Merryshields: The Geese In The Ceiling

Merryshields Journal: 4 Short Stories

Merryshields Activity Book

Kingdom Of Birds

Books by Jennifer Sewell

Adult Fiction

The Time Traveller's Retrieval Service

Links to all books and offerings can be found at www.inkystars.com

ACKnoWLeDGements

As always, many, many people are involved in the birthing of a book. I would like to extend my thanks to all the friends who have supported me, sparked ideas and conversations, been enthusiastic and encouraging, and generally held space for me as I've gone through the various iterations of this book and all the others! This list includes, but is not limited to, the following names: Vanessa Todd, Sunniva Thompson, Elish Mohammed, Hannah Thorpe, Sinead Napier, Becca McPherson, David Jones, Imogen Jones, Eve Jones, Freya Jones, Brodie Jones, Richard Sewell, Elizabeth Aveline, Rachel Bowey-Bland, Elizabeth Sewell, and so many others. I thank you all immensely and heartfully and probably with a big squeezy hug too xxx

www.ingramcontent.com/pod-product-compliance
Lightning Source LLC
Chambersburg PA
CBHW071616030726
47598CB00001B/301